Care

LOUHORUN

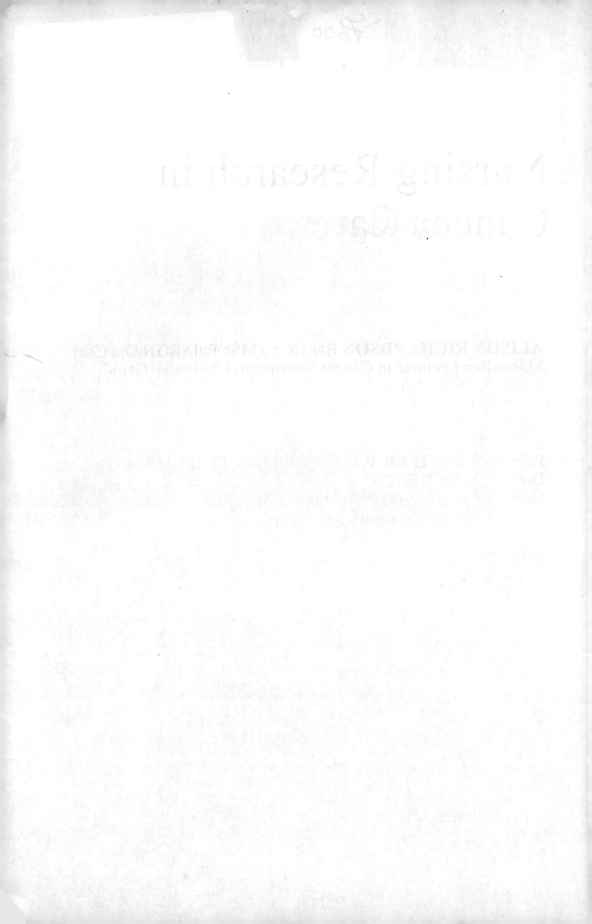

Nursing Research in Cancer Care

Edited by

ALISON RICHARDSON BN(Hons) MSc PhD RGN OncCert
Macmillan Lecturer in Cancer Nursing and Palliative Care
King's College, University of London.

and

Professor **JENIFER WILSON-BARNETT** BA MSc PhD
DipN SRN RNT FRCN
Head of the Division of Nursing and Midwifery
King's College, University of London.

with 18 Contributors

SCUTARI PRESS
London

First published 1995

British Library Cataloguing in Publication Data

Richardson, Alison
  Nursing Research in Cancer Care
  I. Title II. Wilson-Barnett, Jenifer
  610.73698072

  ISBN 1-873853-33-5
Typeset by CBS, Felixstowe, Suffolk
Printed by Bell and Bain Ltd., Glasgow

Contents

Contributors   vii

Foreword   ix
Jeanette Webber

1   A review of nursing research in cancer and palliative care   1
     Alison Richardson and Jenifer Wilson-Barnett

Section 1 Standards and Role Evaluation in Cancer Care

2   Describing breast care nurses   27
     Ann Tait

3   The two worlds of the Macmillan nurse tutor: contrasts and conflicts   49
     Rachel Herring, Stephen J Ball and Jenifer Wilson-Barnett

4   Creating a 'seamless web of care' –   67
     the work of paediatric oncology outreach nurse specialists
     Sarah Bignold, Alan Cribb and Stephen J Ball

Section 2 Culture and Society: Implications for Practice

5   The absent minority: access and use of palliative care services by   83
     black and minority ethnic groups in Leicester
     Hifsa Haroon Iqbal, David Field, Hilda Parker and Zafar Iqbal

6   Policy issues and provision of cancer services   97
     Sue Hawkett

7   A case study of the early detection of cancer in the older adult   113
     Catherine Evans and Alison Richardson

Section 3 Cancer and Personal Relationships

8   The experiences of families of newly diagnosed cancer patients –
    selected findings   137
    Hilary Plant

9   Nurses and involvement in palliative care work   151
    Katherine Froggatt

Section 4 Emotional Reactions and Communication Issues

10 Emotional disclosure between cancer patients and nurses   167
    Anne Lanceley

11 A comparative study of psychological morbidity in women with screen
    detected and symptomatic breast cancer   189
    Alison Farmer, Sheila Payne and Gavin Royle

Section 5 Physical problems: Consequences for Nursing Care

12 The palliative management of fungating malignant wounds:
    preparatory work   207
    Patricia Grocott

13 The pattern of fatigue in patients receiving chemotherapy   225
    Alison Richardson

14 Progress to date   247
    Jenifer Wilson-Barnett

Index   253

Contributors

Professor Stephen J Ball BA(Hons), MA, PhD
Centre for Educational Studies, King's College, University of London.

Sarah Bignold RGN, BSc(Hons), MSc
Research Officer
Centre for Educational Studies, King's College, University of London.

Alan Cribb BA(Hons), PhD
Lecturer in Ethics and Education
Centre for Educational Studies, King's College, University of London.

Catherine Evans BSc(Hons) Community Nursing, RHV, DN, RGN, OncCert
Health Visitor
Camden and Islington Community NHS Trust.

Alison Farmer RGN
formerly Research Nurse
Department of Surgery, Royal South Hants Hospital, Southampton.

Dr David Field BA, MA, PhD
Professor of Sociology
University of Ulster at Jordanstown.

Katherine Froggatt BSc, RGN
Postgraduate Research Student
School of Education and Health, South Bank University, London.

Patricia Grocott BSc(Hons), RGN, DipN
Postgraduate Research Student
Department of Nursing Studies, King's College, University of London.

Sue Hawkett MSc, RN, RSCN, RM, DipN(Lond), CertEd, RNT
Nursing Officer Department of Health.

Rachel Herring BSc(Hons), RGN, OncCert
Research Officer
Centre for Educational Studies, King's College, University of London.

Hifsa Haroon Iqbal
formerly Project Coordinator, Fosse Health Trust, Leicester; now practice Charter
Coordinator, Staffordshire Medical Audit Advisory Group, Stafford.

Dr Zafar Iqbal DCH, MRCGP, MFPHM
Consultant
Department of Public Health Medicine, South Staffordshire Health Authority.

Anne Lanceley BA(Hons), RGN, DipN, OncCert
Senior Lecturer, Head of Cancer Care Studies
The Centre for Cancer and Palliative Care, Institute of Cancer Research, in
association with The Royal Marsden Hospitals NHS Trust

Hilda Parker BA(Hons), CQSW
Research Associate
Department of Epidemiology and Public Health, School of Medicine, University of
Leicester.

Dr Sheila Payne PhD, RGN, DipN
Lecturer in Psychology
University of Southampton.

Hilary Plant RGN, BA
Postgraduate Research Student
Centre for Educational Studies, King's College, University of London.

Alison Richardson BN(Hons), MSc, PhD, RGN, OncCert
Macmillan Lecturer in Cancer Nursing and Palliative Care
Department of Nursing Studies, King's College, University of London.

Gavin Royle MS, FRCS
Consultant Surgeon
Royal South Hants Hospital, Southampton.

Ann Tait MA, RGN, OncCert, DipCounselling
Macmillan Nurse Researcher.

Professor Jenifer Wilson-Barnett BA, MSc, PhD, DipN, SRN, RNT, FRCN
Head of the Division of Nursing and Midwifery, King's College, University of
London.

Foreword

The publication of the NHS R&D Priorities for Cancer Research (1994) heralded a new era for nurses engaged in, or concerned with, research in the field of cancer care. The document sets out a radical cancer research agenda with a strong emphasis on two areas which have always been of major concern to nurses. The first is a focus on the human response of patients and families to the disease, rather than on the disease itself. The second is an emphasis on the development and evaluation of services and interventions which modify the impact of the disease and it's treatment on the individual and family. The chapters in this book reflect these concerns and, at the same time, demonstrate the immense progress made in an important nursing specialty.

Although these works were gathered from the King's College Annual Cancer Nursing Research Conference, the accounts included here are much fuller, with a comprehensive review of relevant literature and specific research approaches. Thus this book provides up-to-date information on key issues as well as insight into the range of projects carried out by nurses.

There are several distinguishing features which unite this work. Not only are the topics relevant to patients' needs, but also the research approaches are eclectic, many methods being employed to answer quite different questions. Increasingly one realises that nurses can achieve so much in research through their willingness to adapt to the situations of data collection by, for instance, asking delicate or sensitive questions at interview, or, in contrast, by applying complex statistical tests, as well as drawing on a broad knowledge-base.

Investment in research and nurses' academic preparation for this work in areas of advanced practice seem to be paying off and the publication of these chapters should provide further impetus in this direction.

This is a very timely book which should make a major contribution, not only to the cancer nursing literature, but also to the nursing literature in general.

Jeanette Webber
Chief Nurse
CANCER RELIEF MACMILLAN FUND

Chapter 1
A Review of Nursing Research in Cancer and Palliative Care
Alison Richardson and Jenifer Wilson-Barnett

Introduction

Recently there has been a rapid increase in the number of research studies carried out in the field of cancer and palliative nursing. This enabled us to capture in this volume an exciting collection of work currently being undertaken by nurses investigating all areas of practice. In reality, the contributors consisted of researchers in the UK that the editors had met through their contacts at the annual research conference at King's College, London.

These current studies have obviously been developed from the knowledge of previous work and we thought it might be useful first to provide a brief review of studies published in the previous five years in order to set the scene. Many of the main categories of research topics are represented in this group, but the directions, focus and method of approach have changed more recently. Within the five years the shift towards more practice-based research is continuing and substantial evaluation and patient-focused work is now evident.

Scope of the Review

This review is provided to give a profile of UK-published research in the last five years, from 1989 to the beginning of 1994. We hope to address the development of research and group work in broad topic areas, to describe the type of studies carried out and identify where gaps exist. Following convention, a computer search of the Cumulative Index to Nursing and Allied Health Literature was carried out. However this search was limited in its ability to identify work which originated in the UK, necessitating an additional search. A manual approach was adopted for this. Major refereed journals for nursing accessible to most practitioners were

1

Table 1.1 Service evaluation studies: Multidisciplinary and consumers' views

Author and Journal	Aim	Design	Procedure and Instruments	Analysis	Findings
Hockey (1991) Nurse author Specialist Journal	To evaluate the extent services were meeting needs	Descriptive, retrospective case reviews on patients who had received home care in previous 10 years. GP and DN questionnaires. Patient, carers, hospice and home care staff interviews	Postal questionnaire Interviews	Frequency estimations	Weakness in communications. Need for earlier referrals to palliative care
Hutchison, Addington-Hall, Bower, Austen & Coombes (1991) Multi-professional authors Specialist Journal	To identify areas of dissatisfaction with the existing service and to make recommendations about how the care provided by the multidisciplinary team might be improved	Descriptive survey. Convenience Sample of n = 93 patients attending a twice-weekly cancer outpatient clinic	Investigator constructed questionnaire	Frequency estimations	Most patients were highly satisfied with the care and information provided by doctors, nurses and other professionals. Dissatisfaction was expressed with the amount of information given about treatment trials and research and with waiting times in clinics and pharmacy. The team was shown to be relatively poor at identifying depressed patients and offering them appropriate services
Inman (1991) Nurse author General Journal	To elicit the child's view of the service provided in a children's oncology clinic	Descriptive, utilising an anthropological approach. Convenience Sample of n = 10 children over the age of 5 years attending an oncology clinic	Audiotape recording of each child and participant observation during two clinic appointments and direct observation of gaze direction of the child and doctor every 15 seconds. Interviews with child and parents separately prior to appointment in the home	Grounded theory was used to analyse the children's and parents' interviews Ethnographic and numerical analysis of material collected during clinic visits	The medical interview was not acknowledged as being very significant by the children: their conscious attention centred on peers and play activities. Clinic visits are more acceptable for children when staff invest personal attention, give appropriate adequate explanations and handle children sensitively
Field, Dand, Ahmedzai and Biswas (1992) Multi-professional authors Specialist Journal	To examine the contact and experiences of lay carers with community nurses and medical practitioners prior to the admission of the terminally ill patient to a hospice, during stay in hospice and following patient death	Descriptive. Convenience Sample. Phase 1 Relatives or carers of patients admitted to a hospice (one week following admission) n= 59, Phase 2 Bereaved carers – interviewed 3 months post death =37	Interview schedule derived from the Life before Death by Cartwright et al	Descriptive statistics including Spearman's correlation coefficient and Mann Whitney U test	Most lay carers were satisfied with the care and attention they received, although they were somewhat less satisfied with the care and attention received from community nurses and GPs than from hospice doctors and nurses. Carers expressed satisfaction with the quality of care received by their relative or close friend as an inpatient and this was an important factor in relieving anxiety
Cox, Bergen and Norman (1993) Nurse authors General Journal	Consumers' perceptions of the Macmillan nurses' work • to identify positive and negative aspects of the role • to test a variation of the critical incident technique	Descriptive case study approach of the work of one Macmillan nurse: 8 randomly selected patients and any associated carers and 5 district nurses and 2 GPs willing to participate. Sample totalled 20	Investigator constructed semi-structured interview (tape-recorded), using a modified critical incident technique	Inductive classification of the information to form categories; the basic unit of analysis was a 'critical happening'.	12 positive and 9 negative aspects of the Macmillan nurse's role emerged as themes by the 4 responding groups. Some themes emerged as important to one or two groups, e.g. availability of the service was a positive feature for patients, while district nurses valued an education element. The Macmillan nurse's specialist knowledge in the area of terminal care and the provision of psychological support were universally acknowledged

included: *International Journal of Nursing Studies, Journal of Advanced Nursing, Palliative Medicine, European Journal of Cancer Care* and *Journal of Clinical Nursing*. The journals were selected on the basis that they are acknowledged to publish research findings and were expected to include a number of cancer and palliative care nursing research reports. Two of the journals selected (*Palliative Medicine* and *European Journal of Cancer Care*) focus specifically on the areas of cancer and palliative care and take a multidisciplinary stance.

Specific inclusion criteria were used for this review. Studies were included in the review if they were published in English by one or more authors in the UK and focused on an area of study directly pertinent to cancer and palliative nursing practice or education. The majority of projects included a nurse as author or co-author; however, a number of projects were included where the sole investigator was not a nurse when the focus of the study was considered extremely pertinent to this review. Clearly, areas such as the evaluation of smoking-cessation programmes have relevance to the specialty, but they were excluded during this review on the basis that they reported on aspects relevant to general health promotion. Similarly, reports limited to the description of quality assurance programmes are relevant to this specialty but were excluded.

Thirty studies resulted from the above search following the application of the inclusion and exclusion criteria and will be included in this review. A substantial number of cancer and palliative nursing studies have been published in the general nursing journals, most notably the *Journal of Advanced Nursing*, representing sixteen papers in total. Six appeared in the *European Journal of Cancer Care*, five in *Palliative Medicine*, four in both the *Journal of Clinical Nursing* and the *International Journal of Nursing Studies* (some studies were reported in more than one journal).

This review is divided into two parts. The first deals with studies classified according to topic areas. This clustering approach allowed the identification of areas in which a number of studies have been completed, where early research activity is evident, or where little, if any, research has been reported. The second part considers the research approach and methods exploited in each area of nursing research. If we have misinterpreted or misclassified studies in any way we apologise in advance!

Assessment of Services

In this area mostly descriptive studies with groups of staff and service-users were reviewed. A growing number of studies are seeking consumer views on services, an encouraging trend in the light of government initiatives, such as *The Health of the Nation: One Year On* . . . (DoH, 1993). Work in this area (see tables 1.1 and 1.2) tends to use interview or questionnaire data to gather views on services used. Retrospective analysis of cases and personnel involved in care is also represented.

Table 1.2 Comparisons between staff's and patients' views

Author and Journal	Aim	Design	Procedure and Instruments	Analysis	Findings
Hunt (1991) Hunt (1992) Hunt and Meerabeau (1993) Nurse authors General Journal	Exploration and comparison of perception and expectations of what constitutes a good death in western society as compared to 5 symptom control team nurses on home visits to terminally ill patients and to describe how nurses gave care	Descriptive. Convenience Sample of 5 symptom control team nurses and their visits to 54 terminally ill cancer patients and their families	Audiotapes of nurses', patients' and relatives' conversations	Case study approaches and ethnographic theories were used for the analysis of conversations	Perceptions and expectations were termed 'scripts' for dying. The elements of the scripts for a 'good death' were identified as: a) control of physical symptoms b) acceptance of cancer and its prognosis, preservation of hope and will to live c) mobility and fighting back d) enjoyment of life e) peaceful death at home
Bergen (1992) Nurse author General Journal	a) to establish the extent to which needs-based criteria laid down in the Health Authority Standard on Care of the Dying were satisfied in the view of district nurses b) to establish the extent to which the stated objectives and Standard criteria were satisfied in the view of the continuing care nurses. c) to establish the extent of the relationship between nursing assessment/intervention and the patient's perception of his/her need	Descriptive multiple case study. Convenience Sample of 9 patients (3 from each continuing care nurse's caseload) and their visiting district nurse and continuing care nurse, totalling 27 interviews in all	Investigator constructed interview schedules for patients, district nurses and continuing care nurses asking practitioners whether they considered the criteria of the standard to be fulfilled and patients whether they felt their needs had been met. District nurse/ continuing care nurse questionnaire relating to standard setting	Content analysis of interview data and utilisation of Yin's approach for within- and cross-case analysis	Needs were felt to be generally well met by the nurses and patients indicated no serious areas of omission. However, a number of recurrent problems and issues was raised. Structure criteria of time, staff, referrals, knowledge and skill and equipment were generally adequately fulfilled and where they were not compensatory mechanisms operated. Process criteria of symptom control and practical care and psychological/ emotional care and support were met to varying degrees by either the district nurse, continuing care nurse or both. Less obvious symptoms such as fatigue were often not picked up. Issues emerged related to the GP and the major role played by the carers other than nurses in relation to certain needs. Outcome criteria of support for carers, preferred place of care and meeting needs were met in the majority of cases. However there was a recurring theme of failure to meet carers' needs

As with many such studies, findings reflected an overall positive evaluation, with substantial satisfaction of those sampled.

A further dimension was added by Hockey (1991) who attempted to reflect the opinions of all those involved in the service through a multidisciplinary focus as well as a consumer sample. In this way, a more critical impression was gained and weaknesses in communication were identified through this work, although most home-care needs were met. General practitioners were also included and not unusually their comments exposed breaches in community–hospital continuity.

It is now quite established from these studies and earlier work that specialist teams tend to win more positive appreciation than other generalist community staff (Cox, Bergen and Norman, 1993; Field, Dand, Ahmedzai and Biswas, 1992). These opinion surveys tend to reveal that the greater amount of time devoted to clients and the increased continuity of care is most appreciated. In contrast, the general areas still receive reports of poor communication and delayed transfers between services.

However, there are exceptions to this trend and perhaps one of the most challenging areas for studies involves outpatient care. For example, evaluation of an oncology clinic using a grounded theory approach with children of over five years and their parents involved observation and taped consultations (Inman, 1991). The medical consultation was not seen by children as the most significant aspect of the visit, their peers and play opportunities were more important features. During this study it was observed that doctors took on a rather dominant role and were frequently interrupted during clinical examinations. Busy outpatient departments may not provide the ideal environment for open and continuous communications during consultations with clients and in general children may present even more of a challenge.

Availability and continuity of services and specialist expertise were seen as essential to all consumers, both patients and their main carers in most research. However, although carers were generally appreciative, in one study there did appear to be a lack of adequate opportunity for them to remain in contact with professional helpers after their family member had died (Field, Dand, Ahmedzai and Biswas, 1992). Some negative comments were also made about communications within the team and between the specialist and generalist teams in these studies.

In some of these opinion surveys on palliative care, comparisons between groups of respondents were also made (see table 1.2) as opinions are known to vary among groups. Evaluations are obviously dependent on expectations of care; work by Hunt in 1991 and 1992 explored differences in views across five specialist palliative care teams and a sample of patients and their families. Taped conversations with consumers revealed many similarities in features considered necessary for a 'good death'. Most mentioned the lack of symptoms and a positive adjustment prior to a peaceful death at home as desirable. When talking to symptom control team nurses about their roles, they agreed with this outcome, but interestingly nurses classified their roles with patients during this period as bureaucratic,

Table 1.3 Nurses' views on the stress associated with carers and cancer care

Author and Journal	Aim	Design	Procedure and Instruments	Analysis	Findings
Copp & Dunn (1993) Nurse authors Specialist Journal	To identify the five most frequent and the five most difficult problems perceived by nurses in the hospice, community and acute care settings when caring for dying patients and their families.	Descriptive survey. Convenience Sample of n = 167 (community = 53, hospice = 53 and acute care = 61)	Investigator constructed open-ended questionnaire sent by post and also handed personally to a number of the sample.	Development of categories by which the data could be coded with main categories subdivided and frequency estimations calculated.	The main categories were physical problems, work-related problems, death-related problems, emotional problems, nurse-related problems, communication, family-related, losses and changed and spiritual problems. Across the three settings the most common problems encountered were physical but were less often perceived as difficult. Nutrition and pain were the two most frequently encountered across the three settings in the physical problems subcategory.
Hanson (1994) Nurse author General Journal	To undertake a theoretical study of the concept of stress applied to persons with cancer as perceived by cancer nurses and to interview and observe nurses to identify areas of perceived stress for patients.	Descriptive approach using phenomenology. Convenience Sample of n = 40 qualified nurses on 4 wards in a regional cancer hospital.	Investigator constructed interview guide. Non-participant observation of 30 nursing admissions. Kardex analysis of 20 nursing assessments.	Content analysis.	Common-sense understanding of the cancer nurse were present in relationship to stress and the person with cancer. Two disparate views regarding stress and persons with cancer emerged: a biomedical approach and a humanistic approach.
Crockford, Holloway and Walker (1993) Multiprofessional authors General Journal	To explore nurses' perceptions of patients' informational, psychosocial and counselling needs, surrounding admission and subsequent breast surgery.	Descriptive, utilising grounded theory approach. Convenience Purposeful Sample n = 8 first and second level nurses from 2 surgical wards.	In-depth unstructured interviews including very broad questions which became progressively more focused.	Grounded theory approach to analysis.	Twenty categories and four theoretical constructs were identified from the data: existential plight, a woman's perspective, being in the dark and patient advocacy. Informants believed breast surgery patients to be very vulnerable and to be suffering from extreme stress and trauma. The phases of not knowing and waiting were seen as particularly stressful.
Corner and Wilson-Barnett (1992) Corner (1993) Nurse authors General and Specialist Journal	To collect baseline information on nurses' attitudes, knowledge, confidence and perceived educational needs in cancer care and test an educational intervention.	Descriptive and three-group quasi-experimental design. Sample of newly-registered nurses' Attitude and Knowledge baseline n = 127. Evaluation of workshop n = 107.	Quantitative and qualitative methods. Pre- and post-assessment using self-report: Cancer Attitude Scale, competency to care scale, knowledge test and interview. Tape-recordings of workshops and observation of seminars.	Quantitative: examining for differences between research groups and within groups and over time. Qualitative content analysis of interviews and tape-recordings of educational workshops.	Baseline study. Perceived competence to care for cancer patients: newly registered nurses rated themselves as most competent in giving physical care and least competent in specific areas of communication and psychological care. Following workshops, nurses rated higher on knowledge and perceived confidence.

biomedical, social, or friendly/informal, apparently altering their approach. These altered according to the problems or stage of the illness.

Some of these findings were mirrored in a study by Bergen (1992) using case studies to assess the extent that needs were met according to pre-set criteria for dying patients. Patient, carer and staff interviews showed overall agreement on care provided. Patients' needs were usually met, apart from a few serious omissions. Carers' needs, however, were frequently found to be unmet. This therefore seems to provide a focus for more study and practice development.

Staff's Opinions and Roles

Perhaps not surprisingly, there were more papers in this category than any other. Ease of access to samples may well account, in part, for this. Studies included explored the experience of caring for those with cancer, identifying by interviews the most stressful aspects of this both for patients and staff and for all employed. For instance, Copp and Dunn's (1993) interviews with nurses aimed to identify the five most difficult problems for hospice and acute care nurses. They found the most common problems were physical, yet these were not seen as the most difficult to resolve. Although there was a wide range of problems mentioned by nurses, the most unmanageable were associated with patients' difficulties in adjusting to their terminal status and separation from their families.

Recent work by Hanson (1994) using a phenomenological interview and observational approach explored areas of stress perceived by nurses on behalf of patients. Feelings of loss, helplessness and worries about remaining family members were frequently experienced. Fears of the unknown and of suffering were also uppermost. Despite an espoused aim to search for a more coherent model of stress applied to this area, the researcher was foiled by nurses who used a 'common-sense' understanding of stress.

Another qualitative interview study (Crockford, Holloway and Walker, 1993) on an in-depth and small scale explored nurses' views of psychological care needs for those having surgery for breast cancer. 'Inadequately prepared' and 'extremely vulnerable' epitomised how nurses perceived this group of patients. All nurses experienced an obligation to act as advocates for these patients and admitted a close identification with them. Recognition of unmet need and inadequate support emerged.

Nurses' own vulnerabilities and fears were also studied by Corner and Wilson-Barnett (1992) in an education intervention study. This was, in part, stimulated by the realisation that patients' needs cannot be met if nurses have deep-seated ambivalence in this area. Although the intervention workshops were not particularly effective at changing long-term attitudes, knowledge and confidence were found to be increased after three months. In-depth interviews and attitude scales were employed by the team and revealed an initial profile similar to that expected in the general population. Nurses were unrealistically pessimistic about treatment

Table 1.4 Nurses' communications and roles

Author and Journal	Aim	Design	Procedure and Instruments	Analysis	Findings
May (1993) Non-nurse author General Journal	Exploration of a range of aspects of the nurse-patient relationship, using the issues raised by terminal care as a mediating question.	Descriptive, using Strauss' methodological theory. Convenience Sample of n = 22 staff nurses with > 2 years' experience.	Investigator constructed semi-structured interview.	Qualitative constant comparative analysis.	Nurses characterised themselves as marginal actors in decision-making about confirming a lethal diagnosis, but expressed a general preference for open and honest disclosure. The lack of concrete clinical criteria on which patients should be told and the practical, ethical dilemmas that disclosure involves added to the stress reported in decision-making about disclosure.
Wilkinson (1991) Nurse Author General Journal	To identify: a) the extent to which nurses use facilitating and blocking behaviours when communicating with cancer patients; b) if there is a relationship between the extent to which nurses use blocking or facilitation and their attitudes to death; c) Nurses' awareness and views about communication patterns.	Descriptive analytical relational survey. Convenience Sample of n = 54 nurses working on the selected wards in a specialist cancer hospital and general hospital.	Self-administered questionnaire which included Collet & Lester's Fear of Death Scale Norbeck Social Support Questionnaire Spielberger State Trait Anxiety Scale. Tape-recorded history. Interviews on difficulties in caring for patients. Field notes.	Tape-recorded nursing histories were transcribed and rated by two independent psychologists for: a) whether each verbalisation was facilitative or blocking in nature; b) rating of whether a nurse covered seven key areas. Interviews and questionnaires.	The findings indicated an overall poor low level of facilitative communication, with a patient's recurrence causing the most difficulties. The coverage scores were low for the key areas and in total. They were particularly low in the area of psychological assessment in comparison with physical assessment. Analysis of verbal behaviours revealed that nurses use different styles of communicating while conducting a nursing history; the facilitator, the ignorer, the informers and the mixers.
Whale (1993) Nurse author General Journal	To explore and describe the participation of nurses in a weekly multidisciplinary ward round and to identify nurses' contributions to and views of those ward rounds.	Descriptive. Convenience Sample of 13 multidisciplinary meetings prior to meeting a patient and 3 multidisciplinary group meetings, yielding a sample of 12 nurses participating in ward rounds on 23 occasions.	Investigator constructed interview to elicit nurses' perceptions of ward rounds. Non-participant observation of ward.	Qualitative content analysis of verbal contributions to round, post-round interviews. Quantitative frequency estimations of nurses' contributions.	Nurses contributed verbally to 81% of the patient cases. The nurses' contributions covered such areas as signs and symptoms, psychological status, social circumstances and discharge planning. Information needs were infrequently raised.
David (1993) Nurse author Specialist Journal	To explore the concept of rehabilitation as a team activity in the oncology setting. Teamwork and rehabilitation.	Descriptive utilising a grounded theory approach Purposive Convenience sampling to reflect members of the multidisciplinary team n = 15	Semi-structured tape-recorded interviews/observations in the form of field notes.	Transcription of tapes, followed by generation of codes which were applied to phrases/words, then grouped into categories reflecting focus of emerging theory.	Staff recognised the existence of team and sub-teams, which interacted in networks of care, communication and patient referral. Teams were seen as fluid, with merging and changing borders. The essence of rehabilitation was seen as the facilitation of the patients to become self-caring and to attain an optimal quality of life.

success and expressed very deep and unresolved fears about their own mortality (see table 1.3).

Obviously nurses' beliefs and attitudes will affect their relationships with patients, as well as their communications and their roles within the team (four studies in this area are described in table 1.4). In May's (1993) study with 22 fairly experienced nurses, they expressed a preference for open and honest disclosure. However, their marginal status in decision-making caused dilemmas and they lacked the opportunities to influence policies for care. Lack of clarity on related policy from medical staff caused distress for these specialist nurses. Related work by Wilkinson (1991) aimed to describe nurse–patient interaction by analysing tape-recorded nurse–patient interaction and found a poor level of facilitative communication, with examples of nurses blocking and diverting conversations. They themselves reported that dealing with those patients admitted with recurrence was seen to be the most challenging and difficult situation. Nurses' personal attitudes to death and a particular ward atmosphere were found to be associated with certain patterns of communication. Positive attitudes and a supportive environment encouraged more supportive communications.

Such findings may well be related to how nurses give care and function in clinical settings. In some situations professional communications among the team may also reflect the attitudes, confidence and knowledge of various groups of staff. For example, in a general setting when studying the nurses' role in multidisciplinary group meetings and ward rounds, Whale (1993) found that while nurses reported their observations on a majority of patients they tended to be reactive within the team, in contrast to medical members. However, greater experience within the specialty seemed to influence the nurses' contribution. 'Teamwork' within the team was also explored by David (1993) in specialist areas where a much more positive and cohesive view of teamwork in rehabilitation emerged. Staff recognised the existence of a team as fluid with changing roles in order to facilitate rehabilitation.

From reading these studies one realises that researchers are really trying to gain new insights into the factors which affect care. In-depth interviews coupled with observation studies achieve a fuller picture than single-method, the approved method adopted in earlier studies. Concern over the quality of communications and openness is now plentifully documented and nurses in particular seem aware of problems occurring in communication. The subjugation of nurses to medical staff in the less-specialised units is also not surprising and may reflect less experience, as well as unresolved and often disproportional fears of death associated with cancer.

Patients' Experience of Cancer

In the last five years three studies in this area were identified: two using qualitative methods (discussed initially) and one a more quantified data collection (see table 1.5). In Payne's study of women with advanced cancer, factors which affect

Table 1.5 Patients' experience of cancer

Author and Journal	Aim	Design	Procedure and Instruments	Analysis	Findings
Payne (1990) Nurse author General Journal	To investigate the factors associated with psychosocial distress in women with advanced cancer	Descriptive using a grounded theory approach. Convenience Sample of n = 24 patients with breast and ovarian cancer receiving palliative chemotherapy either at home or in hospital (subsumable from larger study)	Investigator constructed semi-structured interview covering the areas of previous cancer treatments, effects of chemotherapy on current lifestyle, marital and social relationships, psychological coping responses and perceptions of health professionals' and patients' interactions	Grounded theory approach	The women used a complex range of coping strategies which varied from active problem-solving techniques such as seeking additional information, to strategies that reduced threat such as minimisation and selective attention. In the main the latter strategies were predominantly favoured. The main hypothesis proposed as a result of the study was that patients cope with palliative chemotherapy using four characteristic approaches: think positive/fighter, acceptance, fearfulness and hopefulness. They provide important indicators of communication preferences and informational needs
Faithfull (1991) Faithfull (1992) Nurse author General Journal	To record the experiences of adult patients with a brain tumour after having completed radiotherapy and to establish if somnolence syndrome existed and was a problem for patients	Descriptive. Convenience Sample of n = 12 patients who had completed a course of cranial radiotherapy	Investigator constructed self-report diary completed daily for 6 weeks (visual analogue scales and open-ended items) Semi-structured interview post-diary completion	Qualitative analysis of interview to develop a description of the phenomenon. Visual analysis and construction of confidence intervals to establish where change occurred	Patients experienced a phase of sleepiness which they described as 'exhausted doing nothing' and that any activity was a struggle. Two distinct stages of symptoms were identified, the first occurred on average from day 13 to day 26, the second a distinct period on average between day 32 and day 36. Some individuals described sensory changes, deafness and an increase in leg and arm weakness. Most participants described it as a mental rather than a physical feeling
Corney, Everett, Howells and Crowther (1992) Non-nurse multi-professional authors. General Journal.	To investigate the psychosocial and psychosexual adjustment of women following major gynaecological surgery for cancer	Descriptive. Convenience Sample of n = 105 women who had major gynae surgery in a previous 5 year period (76% of total sample possible). Unclear if and when partners' responses included in sample, partners' responses mentioned in results	Investigator constructed interview schedule, content not specified. Hospital Anxiety and Depression Scale	Frequency estimations	A high proportion of women were found to still be depressed and anxious and the majority reported chronic sexual problems. A high proportion would have liked more information of the after-effects of the operation, including physical, sexual and emotional aspects. Many women would have liked their partner included in discussions. Women also indicated need for emotional support, discussion and counselling

distress and modes of coping were explored. The rich data collected gave indications for the types of support required and ways in which these might be assessed. Hospital and home interviews provided opportunities for in-depth interviewing. Likewise Faithfull's (1991; 1992) study reports that interviews were more successful if both settings were used. This work examined the experience of post-radiotherapy somnolence. Sensitive interviewing and probing achieved a complex yet distinct pattern of symptoms which emerged about this phenomenon.

In a more quantitative study, Corney, Everett, Howells and Crowther (1992) used psychometric scales and structured interviews to detect the level of psychological morbidity among women with gynaecological cancer. As with previous research, high levels of morbidity were detected, compounded by a felt lack of information and a perceived need for more support and counselling.

Thus studies with different research approaches seem to produce findings of a similar nature. Substantial distress is associated with cancer and treatment. More understanding of this is gained through open and in-depth interviews and the courage and sensitivity of researchers to discuss such fundamental issues with patients must be acknowledged. However, the more research reflects these experiences, the more one realises the extent of need for psychological support. Needs seem so prevalent that all staff must somehow be prepared to provide psychological care. Constraints revealed in practice settings by studies in the previous section where staff admit and discuss their limitations give cause for great concern, particularly when linked to the immense unfulfilled level of need.

Physical Problems: Assessment

This section spans the methods used to assess needs and the findings of studies relating to responses to physical treatments. Fewer publications in the area of physical care needs were found, which was not surprising. It represents a previously observed trend; psychosocial studies have always been more numerous (Wilson-Barnett and Richardson, 1993). Hopefully more work will develop, perhaps based on some of the more qualitative work exploring the experiences of cancer and treatment (both psychological and physical) such as that by Faithfull (1991; 1992, mentioned in the previous section).

Three papers by Holmes and colleagues (1989-93) aimed to evaluate the validity, reliability and use of an adapted McCorkle and Young Symptom Distress Scale (see table 1.6). This painstaking work demonstrates the value of a programme of studies building on previous research and expertise. This rigour in testing has produced a valuable tool with great potential for further research and practice.

A fourth study (Sutcliffe and Holmes, 1991) explored the construction and testing of a Quality of Life Scale for cancer patients. Such a useful instrument, tested across hospital populations, could really support further work and in particular meets the need for a sensitive outcome measure for evaluation research.

Table 1.6 Physical problems: assessment

Author and Journal	Aim	Design	Procedure and Instruments	Analysis	Findings
Holmes (1989) Nurse author General Journal	Evaluation of the validity and reliability of a modified symptom distress scale which would permit comparison between patients and between subgroups within a sample population	Methodological Study. Convenience Sample of n = 120 cancer patients admitted to a regional oncology unit	Completed an adaptation of the McCorkle & Young Symptom Distress Scale	Estimates of validity and reliability including Cronbach's alpha, correlation matrices, forward stepwise multiple regression, principal components analysis	Reliability of the tool was high, Cronbach's alpha was 0.97. Most of the items had statistically significant zero order correlations suggesting that most symptoms were closely interrelated and contributed significantly to the total symptom distress score and this was supported through the principal components analysis. Scale was as effective as and easier to administer than the original
Holmes and Eburn (1989) Nurse authors General Journal	To compare nurse ratings and patient ratings of symptom distress	Descriptive. Convenience Sample of n = 53 cancer patients and the nurses caring for them	An adaptation of the McCorkle & Young Symptom Distress Scale completed simultaneously by patients and nurses caring for these patients	Frequency estimations, Cronbach's alpha estimation, correlation matrices and student t-test	Although nurses appeared to be able to estimate the degree of distress due to changes in mobility and appearance the presence of diarrhoea, constipation and tiredness they were less effective in perceiving the degree of distress due to the less 'visible' symptoms such as pain, anorexia, nausea, sleeping disturbance
Holmes (1991) Nurse author General Journal	To identify any differences in the degree/extent of symptom distress between two hospitalised cancer patient populations	Descriptive. Convenience Sample of n = 51 cancer patients undergoing chemotherapy or radiotherapy	Completed a self-report adaptation of the McCorkle & Young Symptom Distress Scale	Estimating of Cronbach's alpha, correlation matrices and student t-test	Overall symptom distress was similar between the two groups; there was considerable variation in the extent of that distress and the symptoms causing distress between the two groups. Tiredness was the most common complaint. Patients having CT complained of cognitive and mood changes. Those having RT were more troubled by physical symptoms
Sutcliffe & Holmes (1991) Nurse authors General Journal	To evaluate further the reliability and validity of the Holmes & Dickerson Scale in both inpatient and outpatient populations and to compare the two groups to identify any differences	Descriptive. Convenience Sample of n = 120 (60 inpatients and 60 outpatients undergoing radiotherapy)	Completed a self-report Holmes & Dickerson quality of life questionnaire	Estimation of Cronbach's alpha, forward stepwise multiple regression, principal components analysis	The scale was shown to be feasible in both settings and to be both reliable and valid. It was quick and easy to score and demonstrated marked differences between the two patient populations
Holmes & Mountain (1993) Nurse authors General Journal	Evaluation of 3 oral assessment guides in terms of ability to establish oral status and as tools for practice and research	Methodological Study. Random Sample of n = 33 patients with advanced cancer	Simultaneous observer ratings of oral status using Passos & Brand's oral assessment guide, Beck's oral examination guide and Eiler's oral assessment guide	Content validity assessed by reference to literature and expert panel review. Interrater reliability evaluated with correlations	None of the assessment tools proved entirely satisfactory. No significant differences in the assessment achieved by each of the observers and suggests each of the tools are both reliable and reproducible. However similarities existed with regard to total scores, but marked differences were observed with regard to scoring of the categories

Table 1.7 Physical problems: treatments

Author and Journal	Aim	Design	Procedure and Instruments	Analysis	Findings
Adams, Lawson, Maxted & Symonds (1992) Multiprofessional authors Specialist Journal	To compare the efficacy of scalp cooling in patients receiving two different doses of epirubicin	Descriptive comparison. Convenience Sample of n = 24 (part of a larger study comparing the effects of epirubicin against breast cancer at two dose levels), patients being treated with epirubicin for advanced breast cancer	Hair loss was graded by observation 0 = no hair loss, 1 = slight loss, 2 = moderate patchy hair loss and 3 = complete alopecia. Photograph prior to chemotherapy and at 3rd pulse of chemotherapy	Frequency estimations	Scalp cooling was ineffective at a dose of 100mg/m²; all ten patients developed total alopecia after 2 or 3 pulses. Scalp cooling was highly effective at a dose of 50 mg/m²; only 2 out of 14 patients developed total alopecia. Those in the larger study who did not receive scalp cooling developed total alopecia at 50 mg/m²
David (1992) Nurse author Specialist Journal	To collect information on current practice and policy in relationship to syringe drivers: a) provide information on the extent to which syringe drivers used in the in-patient centres; b) record current practice; c) list drugs currently administered by this route	Descriptive survey. Convenience Sample of n = 11 hospices funded by Marie Curie, providing 327 palliative care beds and admissions of approx. 4000	Information on current practice was collected by interview of personnel in the hospices. Review of recording documentation and patients' records (n = 3013)	Frequency estimations	Of the patients' records surveyed 42% were found to have used a syringe driver for a mean of 5.8 days. 100 patients had 2 syringe drivers for a mean of 5.4 days. Duration of use ranged from less than 1 day to 120 days. 18 different drugs were recorded as being used in syringe drivers during study period. The most frequently used were diamorphine, haloperidol, cyclizine and methotrimeprazine. Combinations of two drugs were used most frequently, the most popular prescription being diamorphine and haloperidol

Table 1.8 Patients' information needs and related practice

Author and Journal	Aim	Design	Procedure and Instruments	Analysis	Findings
Rose, Taylor & Twycross (1991) Multiprofessional authors Specialist Journal	To discover which components of treatment were complied with in the long term and to ascertain which ongoing problems were experienced by patients	Descriptive survey. Convenience Sample of n = 33. Cancer patients with stable chronic lymphoedema	Investigator constructed telephone interview questions about modality of treatment and ongoing problems	Frequency estimations	67% continued to moisturise the skin though only once daily, while 97% continued to wear a compression sleeve. Almost 75% carried out the recommended arm exercises and/or used the affected arm for household tasks. The most common continuing problem was finding clothes to fit the swollen arm and about half considered they had reduced arm and hand function and half continued to experience pain
Coughlan (1993) Nurse author Specialist Journal	The aims of the study were to a) identify the knowledge that patients had about their illness, their treatment and the side-effects of their treatment; b) establish if the patient perceived the knowledge that he had as adequate	Descriptive. Convenience Sample of n = 30 patients receiving chemotherapy and with a diagnosis of cancer	Investigator constructed 37-item interview schedule. Content validation by expert nurse	Frequency estimations	The vast majority knew their diagnosis, the number of treatments involved and the purpose of their treatment. Patients displayed a poor knowledge of the potential side-effects of their chemotherapy and of the names of the drugs they were receiving.
Walker (1992) Nurse author Specialist Journal	To investigate the extent to which an information leaflet on MST and complementary methods of pain control could increase knowledge and thus increase pain relief for cancer patients taking MST at home	One group pre-test, post-test quasi-experimental design. Convenience Sample of n = 15 cancer patients taking MST being cared for at home or due to be discharged home	Pre- and post-leaflet semi-structured. Investigator constructed interview schedules (tape-recorded) assessing pain and pain control, knowledge regarding pain relief and information needs pre- and post-leaflet. Home pain diary adapted from a previous study. Leaflet adapted from a previous study	Descriptive statistics including the sign test and frequency estimations. Qualitative analysis of themes and collection of short case histories to gain overview of individual experience	Knowledge regarding pain control was significantly increased by the administration of the leaflet. Pain control also appeared to increase for some patients as a result of the leaflet and this seemed to be due to increased knowledge and subsequent use of complementary methods of pain control. The patients who benefited most from the leaflet were those with moderate pain, because they needed the information and were actively able to use it

The fifth study in this area attempted to establish the best tool for assessing oral status. None of the tools was found to be particularly robust. For this, Holmes and Mountain (1993) utilised an expert panel in order to help establish validity, and their comments should help with further reconstruction of such tools in this important area.

Physical Problems: Treatment

Only two studies were identified in this area, one testing out the efficacy of a treatment intervention and the other exploring views on policy for treatment (see table 1.7). This obviously presents a clear contrast to the emphasis on evaluation of physical treatments in medical publications. Indeed the first study (Adams, Lawson, Maxted and Symonds, 1992) was presented by a multidisciplinary team of researchers, dealing with the distressing problem of hair loss and the success of prevention through scalp cooling. Positive consequences of this work are bound to encourage increase in this practice in more centres.

The second study by David (1992) surveyed the use of syringe drivers for drug administration in the hospice setting. A comprehensive but uncritical picture of the extent and details of use was provided.

Patients' Information Needs and Related Practice

Many studies and reviews have previously identified unmet needs for information and in the review period similar findings are presented. In this particular group of three studies the extent of patients' knowledge and the consequences of this for them was assessed. Failure to tailor information for individuals' needs and in an accessible format is generally found. However, work by Rose, Taylor and Twycross (1991) looked at patients with lymphoedema, assessing the level to which they followed advice on how to deal with this problem. A substantial majority followed advice and were therefore very clear about the recommendations and their supposed value. In contrast when testing information-giving related to unfamiliar subjects seen as less relevant to patients, patients do not tend to retain or understand this (see Coughlan, 1993). For instance, drug names are often lengthy and unfamiliar and many people, professionals included, find these difficult to recall. Information-giving on side-effects may also have been less well carried out.

However, when specific modes of information-giving (desired to meet specific patient needs) are systematically provided and evaluated positive results are usually forthcoming. As in Walker's (1992) small study, an information booklet on MST was found to be most useful in helping patients with pain control and self-care. So although new insights are not really offered through this work, the direct application to this group of patients is a useful extension (see table 1.8).

Table 1.9 Cancer prevention

Author and Journal	Aim	Design	Procedure and Instruments	Analysis	Findings
McKie (1993a) McKie (1993b) Non-nurse author General Journal	To elicit the views of women with regard to the cervical smear test in groups of women who have and have not had this test	Descriptive. Convenience Sample of Discussion group phase: n = 72 (9 groups). Questionnaire phase: n = 302 working-class women selected on the basis of age, a 20-34 year group and 50-64 year age group from 2 local authority housing schemes	Women-only discussion groups within existing community groups debated several topics ranging from definitions of health to the cervical smear test. Open-ended questionnaire with items derived from the analysis of the discussion group data	Qualitative analysis to identify dominant themes in the discussion groups. Frequency estimations of responses to the questionnaire.	In those who had not had a smear test: a) the call/recall system did not invite all women in the screening target group; b) beliefs and attitudes rather than practical problems were cited as major factors for non-attendance; c) women held strong views on aspects of service delivery they would like to see in place. In those who had had a smear test: a) a high proportion of respondents were screened opportunistically; b) negative views of the service concerned fear and embarrassment and the lack of, or inadequacy of, any explanation; c) the positive aspects of the service were staff attitudes, convenience and familiarity; d) understanding of the cytology process and the aetiology of cervical cancer was not linked to the level of (non) involvement in the screening service
Larkin 1993 Nurse author Specialist Journal	To consider health visiting practice and its relationship to health promotion, specifically male health and TSE	Descriptive. Convenience Sample of n = 10 health visitors n = 9 young men	Investigator constructed semi-structured interview focused on knowledge of issues surrounding TSE	Content analysis	Health promotion activity appeared constrained by traditional practice, reinforced by managerial organisation of services. No evidence of a proactive approach to men's health. None of the health visitors had received training on TSE. Male respondents had no knowledge of the health visitor's role and had little knowledge of TC and TSE.

Cancer Prevention

Only two specific studies were located (as exclusion categories eliminated several studies on smoking cessation) which examined issues concerned with screening and early detection (see table 1.9). McKie's (1993 a, b) publications reviewed aspects of cervical smear tests, utilising women's discussion groups and open-ended questionnaires. Problems with the comprehensiveness of the service were found and women who attended had strong views about what was and should be provided. However, the researcher identified some problematic beliefs and attitudes among consumers which might have affected uptake of this screening facility.

A second more worrying (small-scale) study explored the lack of Health Visitor involvement in advocating testicular self-examination. Neither they nor their clients recognised their potential in this area (Larkin, 1993). Evaluation of screening and health promotion is notoriously difficult, but given the importance attached to health promotion by the nursing profession there is an apparent paucity of research in this area.

Summary

The preceding collation and discussion of cancer and palliative nursing research in the UK over the past five years has revealed a number of distinct groups of studies. This review can be compared and contrasted with a series of articles which appeared on the development and current status of cancer and palliative care nursing research in the USA and Canada (Oberst, 1978; Benoliel, 1983; Grant and Padilla, 1983; Degner, 1984; Fernsler, Holcombe and Pulliam, 1984). These were prompted by the realisation that a critical mass of studies was accumulating and it was judged timely to review progress that had been made, together with an evaluation of strengths and weaknesses and with the ultimate aim of providing direction for future endeavours.

There is apparent value in categorising papers to determine trends, as this has revealed similarities with previous analyses, the least common research topics being related to cancer detection and prevention (Fernsler, Holcombe and Pulliam, 1984). Also insufficient attention appears to have been paid to the area of physiological responses to treatment which has been considered a high research priority (Oberst, 1978). There remains a paucity of information on physical aspects of care such as the phenomena of nausea and vomiting, fatigue and dyspnoea and related nursing interventions, phenomena of high priority to cancer and palliative nursing practice. Theoretical, measurement and practical issues need to be addressed in the future and are vital to the successful integration of biological and psychosocial variables within research studies. In addition there is also a lack of systematic examination of patient and family education programmes in relation to cancer prevention, hospitalisation, self-care and adaptation to illness and the impact of these educational programmes on patient outcomes. Interventions which can be easily integrated into nursing practice must be developed and tested.

In distinction from the American reviews, descriptive studies examining differing models of service provision and professional, client and carer perceptions of such services are more prevalent and form the bulk of cancer and palliative care nursing research in the UK. Different models of organisation have been proposed as a result of such studies although rigorous evaluation of their effects as yet have not really been tested.

There is also evidence from this current examination of published work in the UK (although it does not claim to be comprehensive) that a few investigators have instigated programmes of research across a span of years, developing expertise in one area as with the work of Holmes. Apart from this, there is a lack of evidence that substantial programmes of research are in progress. Review of this research has also revealed a lack of any trend towards programmes of work by groups of investigators. This will be necessary in the future if substantial and sustained contributions to the scientific knowledge base of cancer and palliative nursing practice are to result from this research activity. On the present evidence, scattered single studies predominate.

Methodological Considerations

Many differing methodological approaches were employed in this specialist area of research. Some research studies also used more than one method and this may have reflected the multidisciplinarity of the research team as well as a growing appreciation of the value of 'mixed methods' studies.

Table 1.10 Descriptive studies with quantitive data

Copp G & Dunn V (1993)

Corney R, Everett H, Howells A & Crowther M (1992)

Coughlan M (1993)

David J (1992)

Field D, Dand P, Ahmedzai S & Biswas B (1992)

Hockey L (1991)

Holmes S (1989)

Holmes S & Mountain E (1993)

Hutchison G, Addington-Hall J, Bower M, Austen M & Coombes C (1991)

Rose K, Taylor H & Twycross G (1991)

Of the 30 studies reviewed, 10 can be described as descriptive, utilising quantified data-collection methods in order to gain information on the relative frequency of a phenomenon or (much more rarely) attempting to devise more sophisticated methods for measuring these phenomena (see table 1.10). These included the useful surveys with consumers and staff laying a foundation of evidence, on the use and evaluation of services.

Given that some descriptive work classifies and then compares results within the same data set or between studies, it may be seen as slightly arbitrary to differentiate between studies which aim to 'compare' or 'describe'. However, having done this, we found three comparative studies (see table 1.11), all concerned with symptom measurement by Holmes and co-workers. Useful work differentiating symptom clusters in patient groups was enabled through statistical analysis.

As might be expected in this challenging area of research only three experimental/ quasi-experimental studies were found, one of which dealt with nurses and two with patient samples. Difficulties in controlling the environment and factors involved in treatment may account for this low number of studies. Additionally the complexity and as yet only partly explored nature of cancer problems makes experimentation on many topics inappropriate. However, future evaluations of nursing interventions may be possible given the relatively rapid rate of growth in knowledge.

Table 1.11 Comparative and experimental studies

Comparative Studies

Holmes S (1991)
Holmes S & Eburn E (1989)
Sutcliffe J & Holmes S (1991)

Experimental Studies

Adams L, Lawson N, Maxted K & Symonds R (1992)
Corner J & Wilson-Barnett J (1992)
Walker J (1992)

Two of the experimental studies, Corner and Wilson-Barnett (1992) and Walker (1992), combined complementary types of data, with qualitative interviews augmenting evidence from the quantified experimental analysis. This approach of combining data seems to be growing encouragingly, despite the extra effort involved in analysing the extensive information produced and the challenging task of comparing or triangulating findings. Two other descriptive studies employed qualitative and quantitative methods (McKie, 1993 and Wilkinson, 1991), both of which managed to integrate data to strengthen the evidence provided. Increasingly 'outcomes' research is being encouraged (see Hegyvary, 1993) and given the importance of treating symptoms effectively, careful planning and evaluation of interventions are required in this field. However, a clear range of definitions and measurement are necessary prior to experimental work. Previous work with pain provides a model for studying other distressing symptoms as Hegyvary suggests and both theoretical and applied work is required for most of these.

Those research projects using qualitative methods make up the largest category consisting of eleven studies (see tables 1.12 and 1.13), six using solely open, in-depth interviews and five using both interviews and observations or recordings, again confirming the tendency to use multiple methods (or at least two!). A rich variety of methods can, therefore, be found in this group. Although the interview using open questions is by far the most popular, the context, degree of focus and the mixed sets of respondents distinguish them. Given the sensitive nature of the issues, it is not surprising that interviewees are encouraged to use their own words. When more direct modes of data collection, such as observation or tape-recorded interventions, are utilised and subjected to analysis, first-hand evidence can be produced but this can be fairly time-consuming. Critical incidence can thus be valuable in helping to select meaningful data.

Table 1.12 Descriptive studies using qualitative data

Bergen A (1992)

Cox K, Bergen A & Norman I (1992)

Crockford E, Holloway I & Walker J (1993)

$\left\{ \begin{array}{l} \text{Hunt M (1991)} \\ \text{Hunt M (1992)} \\ \text{Hunt M \& Meerabeau L (1993)} \end{array} \right.$

Larkin P (1993)

May C (1993)

Table 1.13 Qualitative studies using combined methods

David J (1993)

Hanson E (1994)

Inman C (1991)

Payne S (1990)

Whale Z (1993)

The degree of structure of in-depth interviews varied substantially from semi-structured to grounded in-depth conversations. Difficulty in presenting accounts is evident from reading these papers. So much data are analysed that inadequate time for discussion on the themes seems to be a problem. The need to publish sometimes seems to prevent full rumination and reflection, something many researchers confirm. However, the value of this work is unquestionable and the contribution of nurses in this area is great, arguably the greatest of any health profession. Ideally, greater utilisation and generation of theoretical propositions should be found in these research reports. This may become more possible with a greater tradition of nursing research.

In the studies combining observation with interviews, although often small-scale, the findings are impressive and seem extremely well founded (e.g. Whale, 1993; Inman, 1991). This approach seems to be worthwhile and harmonious in terms of the origins of the research epistemology and therefore to be recommended in future. Despite the enormity of the task of analysis, further descriptive studies by Wilkinson (1991), Faithfull (1991; 1992) and McKie (1993a/b) used both qualitative and quantitative data in an attempt to gain a reliable and comprehensive picture. These courageous attempts really give added strength to the development of research processes and understanding as the reports of methods for these particular studies provided full details.

Table 1.14 Studies using combined qualitative and quantitative data

⌠Faithfull S (1991)
⌡Faithfull S (1992)
⌠McKie L (1993a)
⌡McKie L (1993b)
Wilkinson S (1991)

Overall the range of methods applied appropriately has enhanced this field of research. Depth of insight is often achieved from descriptive qualitative studies, but the frequency and typology of problems also need to be carefully established. Combining methods is not easy when exploring all types of data and is very time- and intellectually-consuming. It does, however, seem to accord with holistic nursing and the multi-faceted nature of cancer and palliative care.

So this review sets the scene for yet more fascinating research collated here for the benefit of nurses and others, in order ultimately to improve upon the quality of care through greater understanding.

References

Adams L, Lawson N, Maxted K and Symonds R (1992) The prevention of hair loss from chemotherapy by the use of cold-air scalp cooling. *European Journal of Cancer Care* 1(5):16–18.

Benoliel J (1983) Nursing research on death, dying and terminal illness: Development, present state and prospects. *Annual Review of Nursing Research* 1:101–30.

Bergen A (1992) Evaluating nursing care of the terminally ill in the community: A case study approach. *International Journal of Nursing Studies* 29(1):81–94.

Copp G and Dunn V (1993) Frequent and difficult problems perceived by nurses caring for the dying in community, hospice and acute care settings. *Palliative Medicine* 7(1):19–25.

Corner J (1993) The impact of nurses' encounters with cancer on their attitudes towards the disease. *Journal of Clinical Nursing* 2(6):363–72.

Corner J and Wilson-Barnett J (1992) The newly registered nurse and the cancer patient: An educational evaluation. *International Journal of Nursing Studies* 29(2):177–90.

Corney R, Everett H, Howells A and Crowther M (1992) The care of patients undergoing surgery for gynaecological cancer: The need for information, emotional support and counselling. *Journal of Advanced Nursing* 17(6):667–71.

Coughlan M (1993) Knowledge of diagnosis, treatment and its side-effects in patients receiving chemotherapy for cancer. *European Journal of Cancer Care* 2:66–71.

Cox K, Bergen A and Norman I (1993) Exploring consumer views of care provided by the Macmillan nurse using the critical incident technique. *Journal of Advanced Nursing* 18(3):408–15.

Crockford E, Holloway I and Walker J (1993) Nurses' perceptions of patients' feelings about breast surgery. *Journal of Advanced Nursing* 18(11):1710–18.

David J (1992) A survey of the use of syringe drivers in Marie Curie Centres. *European Journal of Cancer Care* 1(4):23–8.

David J (1993) A study of the role of the rehabilitation team. *European Journal of Cancer Care* 2:129–33.

Degner L (1984) The status of cancer nursing research in Canada. *Nursing Papers* 16(4):4–13.

DoH (1993) *The Health of the Nation: One Year On . . . A Report on the Progress of the Health of the Nation.* London: DoH.

Faithfull S (1991) Patients' experiences following cranial radiotherapy: A study of somnolence syndrome. *Journal of Advanced Nursing* 16(8):939–46.

Faithfull S (1992) The diary method for nursing research: A study of somnolence syndrome. *European Journal of Cancer Care* 1(2):13–18.

Fernsler J, Holcombe J and Pulliam L (1984) A survey of cancer nursing research. *Oncology Nursing Forum* 11(4):46–52.

Field D, Dand P, Ahmedzai S and Biswas B (1992) Care and information received by lay carers of terminally ill patients at the Leicestershire Hospice. *Palliative Medicine* 6(3) 237–45.

Grant M and Padilla G (1983) An overview of cancer nursing research. *Oncology Nursing Forum* 10(1):58–67.

Hanson E (1994) An exploration of the taken-for-granted world of the cancer nurse in relation to stress and the person with cancer. *Journal of Advanced Nursing* 19(1):12–20.

Hegyvary S (1993) Patient care outcomes related to management of symptoms. In Fitzpatrick J and Stevenson J (eds) *Annual Review of Nursing Research* 11:145–67.

Hockey L (1991) St Columba's Hospice Home Care Service: An evaluation study. *Palliative Medicine* 5(4):315–22.

Holmes S (1989) Use of a modified symptom distress scale in assessment of the cancer patient. *International Journal of Nursing Studies* 26(1):69–79.

Holmes S (1991) Preliminary investigations of symptom distress in two cancer patient populations: Evaluation of a measurement instrument. *Journal of Advanced Nursing* **16**(4):439–46.

Holmes S and Eburn E (1989) Patients' and nurses' perceptions of symptom distress in cancer. *Journal of Advanced Nursing* **14**(10):840–6.

Holmes S and Mountain E (1993) Assessment of oral status: Evaluation of three oral assessment guides. *Journal of Clinical Nursing* **2**(1): 35–40.

Hunt M (1991) Being friendly and informal: Reflected in nurses', terminally ill patients' and relatives' conversations at home. *Journal of Advanced Nursing* **16**(8):929–38.

Hunt M (1992) 'Scripts' for dying at home – Displayed in nurses', patients' and relatives' talk. *Journal of Advanced Nursing* **17**(11):1297–302.

Hunt M and Meerabeau L (1993) Purging the emotions: The lack of emotional expression in subfertility and in the care of the dying. *International Journal of Nursing Studies* **30**(2):115–23.

Hutchison G, Addington-Hall J, Bower M, Austen M and Coombes C (1991) An evaluation of patients' satisfaction with care provided by a multidisciplinary cancer team. *European Journal of Cancer Care* **1**(1):15–18.

Inman C (1991) Analysed interaction in a children's oncology clinic: The child's view and parent's opinion of the effect of medical encounters. *Journal of Advanced Nursing* **16**(7):782–93.

Larkin P (1993) An analysis of the role of the health visitor in relation to testicular self-examination. *Journal of Clinical Nursing* **2**(2):121.

May C (1993) Disclosure of terminal prognoses in a general hospital: The nurse's view. *Journal of Advanced Nursing* **18**(9):1362–8.

McKie L (1993a) Women's views of the cervical smear test: Implications for nursing practice – women who have had a smear test. *Journal of Advanced Nursing* **18**(8):1228–34.

McKie L (1993b) Women's views of the cervical smear test: Implications for nursing practice – women who have not had a smear test. *Journal of Advanced Nursing* **18**(6):972–9.

Oberst M (1978) Priorities in cancer nursing research. *Cancer Nursing* **1**(4):281–90.

Payne S (1990) Coping with palliative chemotherapy. *Journal of Advanced Nursing* **15**(6):652–8.

Rose K, Taylor H and Twycross G (1991) Long-term compliance with treatment in obstructive arm lymphoedema in cancer. *Palliative Medicine* **5**(3):52–5.

Sutcliffe J and Holmes S (1991) Quality of life: Verification of a self-assessment scale in two patient populations. *Journal of Advanced Nursing* **16**(4):490–8.

Walker J (1992) A study to develop and assess the value of a leaflet on pain control for cancer patients taking MST in the community. *Palliative Medicine* **6**(1):65–73.

Whale Z (1993) The participation of hospital nurses in the multidisciplinary ward round on a cancer-therapy unit. *Journal of Clinical Nursing* **2**(3):155–63.

Wilkinson S (1991) Factors which influence how nurses communicate with cancer patients. *Journal of Advanced Nursing* **16**(6):677–88.

Wilson-Barnett J and Richardson A (1993) Nursing research in palliative care. In Doyle D, Hanks G and MacDonald N (eds) *Oxford Textbook of Palliative Medicine*, pp.97–102. Oxford: Oxford University Press.

Section One

Standards and Role Evaluation in Cancer Care

Chapter 2
Describing Breast Care Nurses
Ann Tait

Introduction

The subject of breast cancer has generally had greater media, public and professional interest than many other cancers. The figures on breast cancer may in part explain why there is such a strong focus for concern. In the United Kingdom the annual incidence of the disease is 29 870 women and more than 15 000 women die from it each year (Cancer Research Campaign, 1994-5). One in twelve women may have this disease and in the age group 35–54 years breast cancer is the commonest single cause of all deaths among women (Cancer Research Campaign, 1991). It is a capricious disease and may recur at any stage of a patient's lifetime, for there is a wide range of manifestation and possible spread of the various cancers that are incorporated in the generic term 'breast cancer'.

Background to the Breast Care Nursing Role

One outcome concerning breast cancer since the 1970s has been increased awareness of the problems that patients with the disease face and, in some instances, what might be done to help. An example of this was that in the late 1970s researchers in the United Kingdom identified some of the unmet needs for psychological and practical support of patients with breast cancer (Maguire, 1976; Morris, Greer and White, 1977). The first breast care nurses were recruited in the mid 1970s, in the hope that they might help alleviate some of these problems.

Evaluation of the Role

Since then, the breast care nurses' work has been evaluated in particular settings. Though few nurses were involved in these projects and these studies have not been replicated, in each case the breast care nurse was shown to have made a significant contribution to patients' well-being. Consequently it is now known and accepted that adequate psychological assessment of patients' needs, using a limited intervention strategy, information-giving, supportive counselling, practical help and referral to appropriate psychological agencies have improved patient outcome. Other possibly influential factors have been facilitation of informed choices and the nurse's personality (Maguire *et al*, 1980; Maguire *et al*, 1983; Watson *et al*, 1988; Wilkinson, Maguire and Tait, 1988; Cotton *et al*, 1991). In one study there was also evidence that a breast care nursing service was cost-beneficial within the National Health Service (Maguire et al, 1982).

Evidence of Continuing Need for Breast Care Nurses

As a result of some of these evaluations, the recommendations of the consensus conference on the treatment of primary breast cancer (1986) were that every health district should have a multidisciplinary specialist breast team, with an appropriately trained nurse as an integral member. Unfortunately, these recommendations have not been fully implemented, despite continuing evidence concerning patients' need for effective support (Fallowfield, Baum and Maguire, 1986; Fallowfield *et al*, 1990; Audit Commission, 1993). The growth in the number of nurses was particularly slow until the late 1980s. Then, the impetus of the National Breast Screening Programme, the support of Cancer Relief Macmillan Fund in 'pump priming' breast care posts and a course in breast care nursing, starting in London, led to more rapid growth.

The pressure to increase the numbers of nurses continues with Cancer Relief Macmillan Fund's Breast Cancer Campaign advocating minimum standards of care for patients with breast cancer, including access to a specialist breast care nurse trained to give information and psychological support (Macmillan Breast Cancer Campaign, 1994). The Royal College of Nursing has also lobbied Parliament to back their support for doubling the number of breast care nurses in the United Kingdom (RCN, 1994b).

Rationale for Study

Despite the recent and continuing interest in increasing the number of breast care nurses, there has been and is a considerable lack of knowledge about how they are developing their role. Consequently, in addition to the useful and important research already quoted, a study was required that shifted the focus of enquiry from patient outcome to the nurses themselves. This research consists of a grounded study into the experiences of the breast care nurses, how they construct their role and the range of activities they undertake. Individual variations among breast care nurses are also explored, including age, educational and training experience and personality, and the relationship of these both to the range of activities she undertakes in her day-to-day work and to the nurse's satisfaction in her role. This is relevant to the development of the role in the 1990s, as potential purchasers and providers of health care look for indicators of what a breast care nursing service might offer, and managers and educationalists as well as the nurses themselves look for indicators concerning appropriate post-registration education.

The aims of the study are to describe breast care nursing, how nurses construct the role and how it relates to:

• The Royal College of Nursing (RCN) Breast Care Nursing Society's job description, incorporating the clinical nurse specialist role;
• Research-based practice;
• Relationships between practice, training, personality and job satisfaction.

The Job Description

The RCN job description incorporated the general activities of the role, including practice identified through research as beneficial to patients. It was widely used as a guide to the principles of the role and was interpreted locally to allow for varying contexts and situations. It provided a credible and relevant framework of enquiry for the subjects of the research as well as the researcher.

Relationship with the Clinical Nurse Specialist Role

The job description also incorporated the general components of the clinical nurse specialist (CNS) role: managing leadership in clinical, consultative, educational and research functions within a specialised area of nursing care, with much of the theory underpinning CNS development coming from North America (Menard, 1987; Sparacino, 1990).

Relationship with Research-based Practice

The need to focus on the utilisation, dissemination and development of research-based practice, previously identified as being effective, was important. Research-based practice has been accepted as the basis of the CNS role, but equally as the basis of the knowledge and competencies expected of any registered nurse accountable for her practice. (Wilson-Barnett, 1984; Department of Health *Strategy for Nursing*, 1989). Consequently assessment of patients' needs, a limited intervention timing of care (with the onus on the patient to contact the specialist nurse following the initial crisis of diagnosis and treatment for primary breast cancer), information-giving, practical help, facilitation of informed choices, supportive counselling and referral to psychological agencies were all topics that required scrutiny.

Nursing reports had also identified problems for patients with the following: breast prosthesis (Simpson, 1985; Anderson, 1988); breast reconstruction (Brown, 1989); chemotherapy (Tierney, Taylor and Closs, 1989); lymphoedema (Badger, 1988); psychosexual problems (Rutherford, 1988); relationships with partners (Northouse, 1990); relationships with children (Issel, Enseck and Lewis, 1990); and radiotherapy (Cawley, Kostic and Cappello, 1990). So nursing activities in these areas and issues concerning the marginality of the role (Thomson and Twomey, 1989) were of interest.

Relationships between Practice, Education, Personality and Job Satisfaction

It was judged that if significant relationships were discovered between practice, education, job satisfaction and personality, the ways in which they affected each other would be likely to have implications for the recruitment and education of nurses as well as their practice. The key function of the clinical nurse specialist was her clinical practice (RCN, 1988), but education for advanced practitioners was critical for the maintenance of standards and the development of practice (DoH, 1989).

Lewis (1980) has suggested that it should be possible to develop and establish personality-based criteria of 'suitability' for particular jobs, based on assessments of nurses who have achieved some measure of success within the profession. Previous research on breast care nursing, funded by the Department of Health, comparing patient outcomes following interventions by specialist breast care, ward and community nurses, had shown that there were differences in patient outcomes related to the variation in care given by different specialist nurses. As the nurses had similar training, it was possible that differences in personality might be a factor in the results (Wilkinson, Maguire and Tait, 1988).

Though there was some knowledge about the stresses of working with cancer patients, less was known about satisfaction with their work (Wilkinson, 1988), yet job satisfaction is of importance for quality of life, levels of work performance, absenteeism and propensity to leave the job (Redfern, 1979).

Construction of the Nursing Role

It was also important in describing breast care nursing not just to look at the individual nurse in isolation from her work setting, but to identify the social factors that facilitated the nurse's construction of her role and how the wider context in which her work was set affected her practice.

Research Design

The variety of methods used in this study are incorporated within an ethnographic framework. Ethnography, stemming originally from anthropology, is now a more general term used by different disciplines in a variety of ways. The common factor is that it aims to study thought and belief and the way that these relate to human action. A characteristic of ethnography is that the researcher hopes to convey the sense that what they describe is the result of their having in some way penetrated the form of life that they study; of having 'been there' (Geertz, 1988). It was felt that this approach was justified because though a decision was taken to write up the project in the third person, the researcher was in some senses an 'insider' who had 'been there' as a clinically-based breast care nurse over a period of many years, her role as a breast care nurse had been evaluated in research projects and she had also been active in the development of the specialty.

The main argument against insider research is that it is inherently biased. However, the risk of bias is possible in all research (Stanley and Wise, 1993). Some of the advantages of researching one's own peer group can be ease of entry, avoidance of some kinds of disruption, prior knowledge of relevant questions and an enhanced capacity to elicit in-depth data (Lipson, 1984). Most importantly though, the credibility and relevance of the research to the subjects/peer group can be enhanced, as can commitment to implementing subsequent recommendations. Though research is often undertaken by those who are practically inexperienced in the field, Hamric (1983) proposed that work regarding CNS roles might best be done by those with relevant clinical and research experience.

When decisions regarding the research design were made, because the researcher was an insider with an acknowledged and inherent bias towards the subject of enquiry, she felt that a variety of methods might best provide a balanced picture as well as reflecting the complexity of breast care nursing. Other reasons for using a range of methods included the need for confirmation and validation between differing kinds of data. As Corner (1991) has commented, multiple methods can reduce uncertainties of interpretation in some cases and increase explanation of both typical and unexpected findings. For these reasons, methodological triangulation, or a variety of approaches, as described by Denzin (1978) was used.

Criteria for Inclusion in the Study

The nurse had to be appointed specifically as a breast care specialist in a National Health Service health district or board, be working in that post at least 50 per cent of the work time, have been in post at least six months before being interviewed and have a continuing role with patients with breast cancer.

The Population of Breast Care Nurses

This was defined as all those who met the criteria and were practising in the UK. It was to this group of people that findings about the study could be generalised. Letters were sent to the 220 Health Districts and Boards in the United Kingdom requesting information concerning the employment of breast care nurses. There was a 78 per cent response rate. Regional nurses and other sources of information, such as the breast care nursing local groups, also identified relevant nurses in Districts or Boards where no reply had been received. One hundred and twenty nurses were identified. Subsequently it was agreed that 110 nurses fulfilled the criteria and they all consented to take part in the study (100 per cent agreement). The eventual sample included 108 nurses, and visits were made to the large majority of them at their place of work during 1991.

Distribution of the Population

Forty of the breast care nurses (37 per cent of the total interviewed), worked in the same Health District or Board as another breast care nurse. So the eventual sample only represented a total of 88 out of a possible 220 Health Districts or Boards. When there were added the two Health Districts employing nurses who were potentially available to the study but could not be included, the total was 90. This meant that, as far as it was possible to tell, 130 Health Districts or Boards (59 per cent) did not employ a breast care nurse.

Selection from the Population

Demographic and personality data might have been obtained by postal questionnaires from all nurses who met the criteria. A representative sample of the population could then have been interviewed. However, it was decided to interview all available nurses, if possible, at their place of work, for the following reasons. Statistical analysis of the personality measure and the job satisfaction scale would be strengthened by having as large a sample as possible, yet the potentially sensitive nature of the personality questionnaire meant that the researcher was strongly advised to administer it personally to each nurse (she was also advised that individual feedback on personality scores should be made available to those who wanted it and she should be accessible to answer queries as and when these might arise).

Because of the time, effort and money spent on travel to each nurse, it was seen as sensible to establish as complete a picture as possible from all the nurses by interviewing them. This view was influenced by the researcher's prior experience as a clinical nurse member of the breast care nursing group, plus her experience teaching and as external examiner on breast care courses, as it seemed that there were considerable variations in nurses' practice. These were not only due to different individual personalities in different work settings, but also to the variety of their previous education and experiences contributing to varied knowledge, skills and attitudes.

It could be argued that the 108 breast care nurses who consented to take part represented a population, rather than a sample, because nurses were not excluded due to sampling considerations. It was decided, though, that those taking part more accurately represented a sample because it was not known if every breast care nurse had been identified by the researcher. Also because the numbers of nurses were growing, many more nurses would have fulfilled the criteria within a short time of the sample selection and the population to whom generalisations would be made consisted of all breast care nurses practising in the UK.

Methods Used

Nurses completed audiotaped semi-structured interviews, a personality profile and a job satisfaction scale. Patient contact records were also scrutinised. Field notes were used to record observations made during visits.

Tape-recorded Semi-structured Interviews

Interviews formed a substantial part of the research because they allowed the researcher to explore greater depths of meaning than could be obtained with other techniques (Polit and Hungler, 1983). This interview was in survey (non-experimental) form, variously used to explore, describe and correlate data. A limitation of this design is that it addresses only data acquired through self-report.

Inter-rater reliability checks to assess the degree of consistency between raters were undertaken for the open-ended questions with response categories developed by the researcher for coding. Agreement between raters was found to be satisfactory (Tait, 1994). The relationships between nursing activities, training, personality and job satisfaction were analysed statistically.

Qualitative Data: Methods of Interpretation

Open-ended questions to which responses of qualitative data were transcribed were analysed using a grounded theory approach (Glaser and Strauss, 1967). In this, by constantly comparing nurses' answers, new categories and relationships between them emerge. The analysis also related to Stanley and Wise's (1993) theories of 'recovering the personal', in the sense of analysing the nurses' everyday personal experiences in the form of stories about their work; the interactionist view that behaviour results from interaction and is therefore socially determined was also integral to the analysis.

The Sixteen Personality Factor Questionnaire

Cattell's 16 Personality Questionnaire (16PF) is a well-validated test based on factor analysis and measuring factors validated against external criteria with a wide range of occupational groups. The nature of the primary and second order factors was also felt to have validity concerning the characteristics required for the development of clinical nurse specialism (Cattell, Eber and Tatsuoka, 1970).

Job Satisfaction

In a review of the literature on job satisfaction Hale (1986) suggested that there was a lack of consensus as to what job satisfaction really was; consequently assessment of job satisfaction lacked clarity. Mueller and McCloskey (1990) suggested that occupation-specific scales were needed. These views may partly explain why the search for an appropriate measure was unsuccessful. Consequently a specific measure for breast care nurses was developed with a sociologist colleague, Judith Aldridge, who had considerable practice in the field. Since this development, Traynor and Wade (1993) have found that few measures investigating job satisfaction had evidence of reliability or validity; however, the reliability and validity of the breast care nurses' scale have been reported (Tait, 1994). Establishing job satisfaction as a variable allowed relationships between breast care nurses' practice, education, job satisfaction and personality to be explored.

Timing of the Study Process

This was not a longitudinal study in the sense that much of the data was gained during one snapshot of time during visits to individual workplaces. From an ethnographic point of view, however, the collection of background data concerning breast care nursing was an inherent part of the researcher's working life over many years within the culture.

The Statistical Package for the Social Sciences PC Version 3 programme was used for the data base and statistical analysis. In order to preserve readability and focus on meaning, the type of statistical test used is not individually reported for any one finding. Where bivariate levels of association are reported, either the non-parametric Spearman's rank order correlation was used when the variables involved were measured at an ordinal or interval level, or the chi-square test was used when variables were dichotomous. Where multivariate levels of association were reported, a multiple regression analysis was employed. All reported findings were significant with the probability due to chance of less than 5 per cent (i.e. $p < 0.05$), and tests were two-tailed where appropriate.

Results

The results of this study suggest that though there were very considerable variations in individual practice and the settings in which nurses operated, there was some cohesion and consistency about the ways in which certain aspects of the role had developed. There was strong motivation for the role from this self-selected group and there was considerable awareness of their privileged position in supporting vulnerable patients at times of such great need.

Snapshot Summary

The 'typical' breast care nurse was hospital-based, but also worked in the community, was employed at an H grade, had been in post for four years, had five O-levels, one A-level, lived with a partner, had an average of two children, drove seven miles to work and was aged 43 years.

The Construction of the Role

The nursing role was mainly developed within the context of the medically and male-dominated acute sector of the NHS, where there was little cohesion or consensus concerning optimum treatments or standards of care. Consequently this called for sensitive and diplomatic construction and negotiation of the work on a continuing basis, establishing credibility from a marginal position with a range of strategies including deference and assertion, especially with surgeons who were often the gatekeepers to the nursing service.

Nurses felt they could develop their role better within the ethos of designated breast clinics and within multidisciplinary specialist teams, as most of their problems occurred with generalist as opposed to specialist surgeons. One-third of the sample were not in specialist teams and they were more likely to continue feeling isolated and peripheral to existing groupings than nurses who were in specialist teams. This was despite the fact that nurses valued autonomy and scored highly on personality factors such as independence, for they also scored highly as team players.

Generally, little appeared to be done by managers to optimise the role; only 15 per cent of nurses had annual performance appraisals and 64 per cent of nurses had never had one in that job. There was little managerial help to aid successful integration into broader aspects of the organisation, yet 72 per cent of nurses were satisfied with their management. Perhaps this was because managers were not yet so involved in the development of the market economy of the NHS as to interfere at the time of data collection, and nurses valued their autonomy very highly; also the large majority of nurses were not hoping to change their careers and proceed further up the NHS hierarchy.

There was considerable agreement amongst the nurses that the main concerns of patients were threats to their mortality, confidence, sense of control and self-esteem and that the role was mainly constructed round these needs. Consequently many nurses felt that delicate negotiation, sensitivity and diplomacy with patients were important and used a variety of strategies to be 'appropriate', friendly and non-threatening while also being professional.

Core Characteristics of the Role

There was general agreement that the core characteristics of the role were to fill existing gaps in the support available to patients, to complement the existing primary carers and to provide continuity of care according to need; also that the timing and frequency with which care was given resembled that of a potentially recurring crisis intervention model with the onus mainly on the patient to contact the nurse following the initial crisis.

Improving General Standards of Care

There was considerable leadership and collaboration with other health care professionals in setting and maintaining standards of care in hospitals and in supporting staff whether in hospital or the community. Eighty-three per cent of nurses had been involved in standard-setting exercises; some were merely at the planning stage, but half of the sample had already been involved in time-consuming but vital consultation exercises and had produced written standards, available for the researcher to see and currently being implemented. During the research visits, professional colleagues volunteered information concerning the breast care nurses' role in improving standards generally. Amongst others, these included link nurses, who were giving substantial support, junior doctors and consultants as well as the ward and clinic nurses. The researcher also read some of the correspondence received from patients and staff thanking the nurses for their work. Nurses also felt that the written standards that were agreed would serve as the baseline against which audit could be undertaken. The results of these procedures would be fed back in the market profiles to the purchasers of services. Given the disparities in standards of care for patients with breast cancer generally, most nurses felt that the National Breast Screening Programme had been a positive influence towards multidisciplinary specialist care and improved standards.

There was a significant association between nurses who were more independent and emotionally adjusted and their greater involvement in raising standards by education of other health care professionals. Perhaps this was not surprising, given the difficulties involved in helping nurses, doctors and others along their journey from novice to expert.

Dimensions of Care

There was considerable consistency amongst nurses in feeling that their main focus was on a holistic, emotionally supportive model of direct care for patients. This model comprised dimensions initially developed by the researcher but subsequently found to be similar to those revealed by Davies and Oberle (1990) in the palliative care setting.

These dimensions included feeling privileged to be in the role and valuing patients as people. 'Connecting' or 'being there' with patients was another dimension whereby nurses initially had to negotiate credibility with patients and others involved in care including a verbal identity, as with how the nurses introduced themselves; visual identity, as with clothing and badges and territorial identity, as with placement and decor of the nurses' workplace. Gaining trust, assessing need and negotiating the nurses' levels of involvement with patients meant that nurses had to learn to 'tune in' and 'tune out' of relationships. It was clear that nurses attached great importance to 'being there' for patients over time, which involved an emotional attachment, whether the nurses' physical presence with the patients was required or not.

Empowering patients meant facilitating them to take more control if they so wished, by nursing activities such as giving information and using counselling skills. The dimension of nurses as women, empowering patients who were also women, was explicitly stated by many of the nurses. However, alongside this acknowledgement of feminist issues there was also ambivalence about the most appropriate strategy for influencing the mainly male medical hierarchies on behalf of the women; feminine guile as well as professional competence were often felt to be useful.

The dimension of 'doing for' patients incorporated the extrinsic, practical and coordinating aspects of the nurses' role. 'Taking over' in this way was clearly an important part of the crisis intervention regarded by the nurses as vital at the time of diagnosis of primary or secondary cancer and subsequent treatments. Despite this practical focus, much of the work nurses reported when connecting with and empowering patients was concerned with helping patients to 'make sense' of what was happening, though this was rarely explicitly stated. It appeared that 'finding meaning', given the increased awareness of the temporary and fragile nature of life, was not only the prerogative of patients but became part of many nurses' lives and there was considerable acknowledgement that the nurses reordered their own priorities in life as well as helping their patients to do so.

Milestones in the Learning Process

There was evidence that in some geographical areas nurses were influential as mentors and role models and had a significant leadership role; for example, nurses in one area appeared to have greater awareness of women's passivity in their lives generally as opposed to this occurring simply in relation to breast cancer; consequently they felt that trying to empower women at times of such great vulnerability was particularly challenging. Nurses in another geographical area gave particular weight to recording a full psychological assessment of their patients. What members of these local groups appeared to have in common was the experience of undertaking a clinical placement with a frequently mentioned and acknowledged local leader.

Networking, especially within active local groups of the RCN Breast Care Nursing Society, was generally valued, as were their national and local meetings. Importance was attached to attendance at specialist conferences and seminars, also to the English National Board specialist breast care nursing course by the nurses who had taken part in it. However, although 52 per cent of nurses had not yet had the opportunity to take this course, only 23 per cent of the total sample felt that they wanted to undertake this in the future, some finding the possibility of training so many years after their lengthy clinical experience in the field quite threatening.

Adoption of the Principles of the Job Description

Many of the principles of the clinical role and responsibilities outlined in the job description appeared to be adopted by the nurses. These included giving patients information, facilitating them to make informed choices, acting as the patient's advocate and sometimes giving practical care relating to breast prosthesis, breast reconstruction and lymphoedema.

A Communication, Assessment and Counselling Framework for Care

Sixty-one per cent of the sample felt that they used a nursing process approach to their work, but only 20 per cent used a named nursing model when planning and implementing care. Some nurses used models specific to counselling, but of these the most commonly mentioned Rogerian model was used by only 11 per cent of the nurses (Rogers, 1959). Despite this lack of specific nursing or counselling frameworks, over two-thirds of the nurses (69 per cent) said they attached importance to a research-based framework for care incorporating particular aspects of communication, assessment of need and supportive counselling, taught by experiential methods with supervised feedback.

Emphasis was attached within this framework to combining skills in communication and counselling with the content of the assessment which included a range of topics such as patients' mood states or sexual concerns. This format had contributed significantly to positive earlier evaluations of the breast care nurses' role (Tait *et al*, 1982). It had subsequently been developed as a training method (Faulkner and Maguire, 1984). Despite nurses' apparent support for this framework, objective assessment of a sample of nursing records suggested that there was less cohesion and consistency regarding nurses' identification of patients' emotional needs such as clinical depression, anxiety states or sexual problems. Such assessments were recorded by only 40 per cent of the nurses, with only one-third of the sample documenting ongoing evaluations of the care given, and only 12 per cent of the nurses used validated self-report questionnaires to identify patients' mood states. Also, the low level of referrals for psychological therapy (the mean number being three per cent of the nurses' caseload of patients), given the known incidence of 20 to 30 per cent of patients with psychological morbidity, was only partly explained by lack of resources or the fact that some nurses were developing their own counselling skills.

Only 31 per cent of nurses said that they explicitly assessed patients' spiritual beliefs or values, but implicitly it appeared that many nurses helped patients as they developed new meanings in their lives. There were significant associations between nurses who had experiential training using the CAC framework and their willingness to assess patients' mood states, sexuality and coping strategies, amongst other topics. There was a significant association between nurses who had undergone certificated training in counselling skills and their willingness to assess patients' mood states and spiritual beliefs. Given these findings, it was perhaps not surprising that though 47 per cent of nurses had undertaken substantive counselling courses, over two-thirds (70 per cent) of the nurses still wanted further counselling training.

Community Liaison

It was generally agreed that though the nurses provided continuity of emotional support when patients were discharged into the community, liaison with the primary health care teams was often ad hoc and fragmented, with many of them not knowing of the nurse's individual involvement. Despite this there was considerable activity in the community educating lay and professional groups and half the sample were involved with 'self-help' groups. There was a significant association between nurses with community training and undertaking an increased number of nursing activities in the community.

Cancer Nursing

Only seven per cent of nurses had undertaken the recognised oncology nursing course, so it was surprising that only 20 per cent of nurses wanted to participate in such training in the future. By the nurses' own admission, giving information about the biological nature of the disease, the effects of the available treatments, the routine facilitation of prophylactic or remedial measures to combat side-effects and the management of pain was often seen as difficult and in several cases was acknowledged to be patchy. Also, though many nurses did give information concerning a variety of resources for patients, others were either gatekeepers or did not have adequate information about local and national cancer support services including literature, help lines or volunteer groups, to pass on to patients.

Nursing Records

Scrutiny of nursing records suggested that though some gave clear guidelines as to the care given, the structure was extremely variable and the content in the majority of cases was scant. The 'invisibility' of many nurses in an organisational sense was increased as they rarely documented their care in the nursing Kardex or medical records. The guidelines on record keeping by the UKCC (1993) are timely.

Clinical Nurse Specialism

There was little explicit awareness of the theories underpinning clinical nurse specialism, though implicitly many nurses were developing some of these principles within their clinical role. Though many nurses had been innovative in educating others and taught a wide range of people including doctors, there was less consistency in their overall development as educationalists and even less in their development as research resources. These findings were due to a variety of factors including large caseloads, variable past experience, variable educational levels, especially the ability to conceptualise the potential of the job, and variable motivational levels to develop and change, with less than a fifth of the sample wanting training specifically related to developing the CNS role. Organisations were not geared to optimise the service.

Research-based Practice

As the rationale concerning the principles of the RCN job description was based on previous research findings about the role, it could be argued that practice related to these principles was research-based. However, the findings of this study concerning aspects of nurses' support for patients' physical, spiritual and emotional needs suggest that research-based practice varied considerably, as did awareness of the need. The majority of nurses felt that their awareness of psychological research had been influential in their own practice. However, though half of the nurses felt they were influenced by research concerning surgical treatment choices, only a third of the sample suggested that research concerning the range of other cancer treatments, their side-effects and management, was also influential. There was a significant association between nurses who had received higher education with first or second degrees and undertaking increased research activity.

Relationships between Practice, Training, Personality and Job Satisfaction

Some of the relationships between training and practice have already been mentioned. Nurses scored highly on personality factors such as leadership and emotional adjustment; these factors were significantly correlated with innovations in clinical and educational practice. Generally, the nurse's profile was that of an assertive, warm but sensitive and diplomatic carer with creativity and imagination, a degree of flexibility and practical innovation, but also some conservatism. Personality scores were lower in political, managerial or business acumen, which might have implications for development of the role within the market-driven health service.

There were several significant associations between personality and nurses' reported practice. Nurses with higher levels of emotional stability said they were more willing to identify and help with patients' emotional concerns than those without such levels. Nurses who identified their personal belief system as humanist were less willing to assess and discuss spiritual issues with patients than nurses who identified themselves as Christians. Nurses who scored highly as tough decision-makers were more likely to make organisational changes in aspects of care such as prosthesis-fitting than nurses who did not score so highly in tough decision-making. Consequently it does appear that personality factors and personal beliefs as well as training may play a part in explaining variations in nurses' practice.

There were significant relationships between job satisfaction and training, such as completion of the advanced breast care course or a substantive counselling course; also between job satisfaction and developing innovative practice, good relationships with surgeons and specialist teams, managerial and peer support and personal beliefs in Christianity, an after-life or that life is in some aspects preordained.

Job satisfaction was high in an absolute sense, despite less than half the sample having access to professional support. These findings support those of Gowshall (1992). The only significant predictors of job satisfaction were age and emotional stability.

Conclusion

Breast care nurses have been located at the juncture between the dominant influences of surgery, psychology and, to a lesser extent, oncology. They are poised between medical and scientific knowledge of the disease and the illness experience of their patients and have to mediate between medical practice and its distressing impact on their patients' lives. In hostile and supportive settings they have had considerable courage and tenacity in developing their role and there are many examples of the ways in which they have improved care.

Need for a Distinctive Focus

The variety of the nurses' work and size of their caseloads were open-ended, presenting seemingly infinite possibilities of improving care in unclaimed territory. Many nurses experienced difficulties developing a distinctive focus, prioritising needs, placing boundaries around the care they offered and between their personal and professional involvement in work.

Though breast care nurses are increasing in number, it is a relatively new specialty with a knowledge base that is still evolving in focus and content. The findings of this study suggest that though the nurses were motivated to develop counselling skills, they were less motivated to develop a knowledge base related to cancer generally and breast cancer in particular. If breast care nurses are to survive the scrutiny of the providers and purchasers of the health service, it seems that they will need to clarify, develop and articulate their service and the levels of expertise at which they operate. A more distinctive focus on the cancer nursing aspects of physical care as well as more clarity concerning emotional and spiritual support are needed.

Implications for the Future

Though a descriptive study does not provide 'hard' evidence of cause and effect, there did appear to be enough indicators in this study to consider their future implications. The study has already raised awareness or added weight to work now being developed by the RCN Breast Care Nursing Society/Macmillan working groups on nursing competencies and nursing records. The findings of the study support the need for the specialist in nursing practice level envisaged in the UKCC (1994) Standards for Education and Practice following registration, and also for the level of expertise envisaged for the evolving role of the Macmillan nurse (Webber, 1993). As work on defining levels of competence is ongoing, the educational recommendations are confined to the particular topics that require knowledge and skills in order to achieve the required levels of expertise.

It is recognised that the availability of suitable courses, time and money for post-registration education and training presents many difficulties. However it is argued that it may be necessary to aim for a 'critical mass' of nurses who are motivated to be appropriately experienced and educated, rather than encouraging a mushrooming of those who, though compassionate carers, are not necessarily motivated nor yet knowledgeable enough to optimise the role.

Recommendations

Need for a Specialist Level of Expertise

Moving from primary practitioner to specialist would require the necessary competencies to achieve the RCN Breast Care Nursing Society's Standards of Care (1994a) and also education in the following:

- Nursing, medical, lay, women's and management perspectives on breast cancer;
- Oncology, including the biological nature of cancer and treatments;
- Interpersonal skills, including communication, assessment, giving information, supportive counselling and psychological referral, crisis intervention, group and telephone work:
- Self-awareness covering spiritual issues such as values and beliefs;
- Teaching;
- Community liaison;
- Research appreciation and utilisation;
- Simple therapies (e.g. relaxation training);
- Leadership/management within the Clinical Nurse Specialist ethos (e.g. management of change, resource management).

As stated by the UKCC, the level of study would be no less than that of a first degree.

Advanced Practitioner Level

It was not clear how many nurses would wish to work towards this. Very few nurses had a degree at Master's level. If those without appropriate education were motivated to obtain it, this level would accommodate some of the nurses already identified as leaders, mentors and role models.

Clinical Grading

The different levels of expertise should be acknowledged by the clinical grading.

Recruitment: Personal Characteristics of the Nurse

Emotional stability, leadership, maturity and at least five years post-registration were important as predictors of job satisfaction and as the most important characteristics in nurses who were innovative regarding education and practice. Though the personality profile would not predict who was suitable for a job, if there was a situation where several candidates were thought to be appropriate, it might be used as one amongst several methods to facilitate choice.

Nursing Records

Nursing records should be used to develop a framework for practice and clinical audit as well as protecting against litigation.

Organisational Developments

- Before breast care nurses are appointed, operational policies for development of the clinical nurse specialist role should receive 'top down' and 'bottom up' commitment from managers and clinicians.
- Regular appraisal and support for continued development of the role within a multidisciplinary context, from service managers.
- Encouragement of a multidisciplinary team approach to management of breast cancer with the nurse as an integral member.
- Availability of pyschological resource people able to provide support and supervision of nurses' caseloads and to receive referrals of patients with complex problems for therapies.

Future Recommendations

It is likely that in future nurses will be required to justify particular aspects of practice, such as clinical decision-making, as well as the effects of such decisions on patient outcomes; consequently more work will be needed in this area.

Acknowledgements

The author gratefully acknowledges the support of Cancer Relief Macmillan Fund for this study; also the help given to the study by Judith Aldridge, Bogusia Temple and Chintha Dissonayake.

References

Anderson J (1988) Facing up to mastectomy. *Nursing Times* **84**(3):36–9.

Audit Commission for Local Authorities and the National Health Service in England and Wales (1993) *What seems to be the matter: Communication between Hospitals and Patients.* London: HMSO.

Badger C (1988) A problem for nurses – lymphoedema. *Surgical Nurse* October, 14–19.

Brown H (1989) Breast reconstruction. *Nursing Times* **4**(8):26–8.

Cancer Research Campaign (1991) *Factsheet 6.1: Breast Cancer.* London: CRC

Cancer Research Campaign (1994-5) *Scientific Year Book.* London: CRC

Cattell R, Eber H and Tatsuoka M (1970) *Handbook for the Sixteen Personality Factor Questionnaire (16PF).* Illinois: Institute for Personality and Ability Testing.

Cawley M, Kostic J and Cappello C (1990) Information and psychosocial needs of women choosing conservative surgery/primary radiation for early stage breast cancer. *Cancer Nursing* **13**(2):90–4.

Consensus Development Conference: Treatment of Primary Breast Cancer (1986) *British Medical Journal* **293**:946–7.

Corner J (1991) In search of more complete answers to research questions. Quantitative versus qualitative research methods: Is there a way forward? *Journal of Advanced Nursing* **16**:718–27.

Cotton T, Locker A, Jackson L, Blamey R and Morgan D (1991) A prospective study of patient choice in treatment for primary breast cancer. *European Journal of Surgical Oncology* **17**:115–17.

Davies B and Oberle K (1990) Dimensions of the supportive role of the nurse in palliative care. *Oncology Nursing Forum* **17**(1):87–94.

Denzin N (1978) *The Research Act,* 2nd edn. New York: McGraw-Hill.

DoH Nursing Division (1989) *A Strategy for Nursing.* London: DoH.

Fallowfield L, Baum M and Maguire GP (1986) Effects of breast conservation on psychological morbidity associated with diagnosis and treatment of early breast cancer. *British Medical Journal* **293**:1331–4.

Fallowfield L, Hall A, Maguire GP and Baum M (1990) Psychological outcomes of different treatment policies in women with early breast cancer outside a clinical trial. *British Medical Journal* **301**:575–80.

Faulkner A and Maguire PG (1984) Teaching Assessment Skills. In: Faulkner A (ed) *Recent Advances in Nursing: 7. Communication*. Edinburgh: Churchill Livingstone.

Geertz C (1988) Works and Lives: *The Anthropologist as Author*. Oxford: Polity Press Blackwell.

Glaser BD and Strauss AL (1967) *The Discovery of Grounded Theory*. New York: Aldine.

Gowshall K (1992) *The Satisfactions and Stresses of Breast Cancer Nursing*. Unpublished MSc thesis, Department of Nursing Studies, Surrey University.

Hale C (1986) Measuring job satisfaction. *Nursing Times* **82**(5):43–6.

Hamric A (1983) Role development and functions. In: Hamric A and Spross J (eds) *The Clinical Nurse Specialist in Theory and Practice*. London: Grune and Stratton.

Issel M, Enseck M and Lewis F (1990) How children cope with mother's breast cancer. *Oncology Nursing Forum* **17**(3):Supplement 5–12.

Lewis B (1980) Personality profiles for qualified nurses: possible implications for recruitment and selection of trainee nurses. *International Journal of Nursing Studies* **17**:221–34.

Lipson J (1984) Combining researcher, clinical and personal roles: Enrichment or confusion? *Human Organisation* **43**(4):348–52.

Macmillan Breast Cancer Campaign (1994) *Minimum Standards of Care for Women with Breast Cancer*. Press Release 16th May. Cancer Relief Macmillan Fund.

Maguire PG (1976) The psychological and social sequelae of mastectomy. In: Howells J (ed) *Modern Perspectives in the Psychiatric Aspects of Surgery*. Edinburgh: Churchill Livingstone.

Maguire GP, Tait A, Brooke M, Thomas C and Sellwood R (1980) The effects of counselling on the psychiatric morbidity associated with mastectomy. *British Medical Journal* **281**:1454–6.

Maguire GP, Pentol A, Allen D, Tait A, Brooke M and Sellwood R (1982) Cost of counselling women who undergo mastectomy. *British Medical Journal* **284**:1933–5.

Maguire GP, Brooke M, Tait A, Thomas C and Sellwood R (1983) The effect of counselling on physical disability and social recovery after mastectomy. *Clinical Oncology* **9**:319–21.

Menard S (1987) The CNS: Historical Perspectives. In: Menard S (ed) *The Clinical Nurse Specialist: Perspectives on Practice*. Chichester: John Wiley and Sons.

Morris T, Greer S and White P (1977) Psychological and social adjustment to mastectomy. *Cancer* **40**: 2381–7.

Mueller and McCloskey (1990) Nurses' Job Satisfaction: A proposed measure. *Nursing Research* **39**(2):113–16.

Northouse L (1990) A longitudinal study of the adjustment of patients and husbands to breast cancer. *Oncology Nursing Forum* **17**(3): Supplement 39–43.

Polit D and Hungler B (1983) *Nursing Research Principles and Methods,* 2nd edn. Philadelphia: Lippincott.

Redfern S (1979) The charge nurse: Job attitudes and occupational stability. *RCN*

Steinberg collection of nursing research **viii**:249.

Rogers C (1959) A Theory of Therapy, Personality and Interpersonal Relationships as Developed in the Client-Centred Framework. In: Koch S (ed), *Psychology: A Study of Science*: pp.205–7. New York: McGraw-Hill.

Royal College of Nursing (1988) *Specialties in Nursing*. London: Royal College of Nursing.

Royal College of Nursing (1994a) *Breast Care Nursing Society Standards of Care*. London: Royal College of Nursing.

Royal College of Nursing (1994b) RCN *Breast Care Lobby*. Press Release 17th May.

Rutherford D (1988) Assessing psychosexual needs of women experiencing lumpectomy. *Cancer Nursing* **11**(4):244–9.

Simpson G (1985) Are you being served? *Senior Nurse* **2**(6):14–16.

Sparacino P (1990) A Historical Perspective on the Development of the Clinical Nurse Specialist Role. In: Sparacino P, Cooper D and Minarik P (eds) *The Clinical Nurse Specialist: Implementation and Impact.* Norwalk, Connecticut: Appleton and Lange.

Stanley L and Wise S (1993) *Breaking Out Again*. London: Routledge.

Tait A (1994) *Breast Care Nursing.* Report for Cancer Relief Macmillan Fund. London: Cancer Relief Macmillan Fund.

Tait A, Maguire P, Brooke M, Faulkner A, Wilkinson S, Thomson L and Sellwood R (1982) Improving communication skills: Standardised assessments for mastectomy patients. *Nursing Times* **78**(51):2181–4.

Thomson L and Twomey M (1989) Caught in the crossfire. *Nursing Times* **85**(48):51.

Tierney A, Taylor J and Closs S (1989) *A Study to Inform Nursing Support of Patients Coping with Chemotherapy for Breast Cancer*. Edinburgh: Nursing Research Unit, University of Edinburgh.

Traynor M and Wade B (1993) The development of a measure of job satisfaction for use in monitoring the morale of community nurses in four trusts. *Journal of Advanced Nursing* **18**(1):127–36.

United Kingdom Central Council for Nursing, Midwifery and Health Visiting (1993) *Standards for Records and Record Keeping*. London: UKCC.

United Kingdom Central Council for Nursing, Midwifery and Health Visiting (1994) *The Future of Professional Practice: The Council's Standards for Education and Practice following Registration*. London: UKCC.

Watson M, Denton S, Baum M and Greer S (1988) Counselling breast cancer patients – a specialist nurse service. *Counselling Psychology Quarterly* **1**(1):23–31.

Webber J (1993) *The Evolving Role of the Macmillan Nurse*. Working Paper. London: Cancer Relief Macmillan Fund.

Wilkinson S (1988) Nursing Patients with Cancer: Satisfactions and Stresses. In: Faulkner A (ed), *Oncology*. London: Scutari Press.

Wilkinson S, Maguire P and Tait A (1988) Life after breast cancer. *Nursing Times* **84**(40):34–7.

Wilson-Barnett J (1984) *Key Functions in Nursing.* The Winifred Raphael Memorial Lectures. Monograph. London: Royal College of Nursing.

Chapter 3
The Two Worlds of the Macmillan
Nurse Tutor: Contrasts and Conflicts

Rachel Herring, Stephen J Ball and
Jenifer Wilson-Barnett

Background

The primary aim of the research reported here was to explore the work activities and institutional roles of the Macmillan nurse tutor (MNT). MNTs are specialist tutors responsible for palliative and/or cancer care education. The underlying aim of these posts is to improve patient care through the education and professional development of nurses and to raise the profile of cancer and palliative care. All such tutors have links with both a College of Nursing and a clinical area, for example a hospice, although the exact nature of these links varies. Cancer Relief Macmillan Fund (CRMF) pump-prime these MNT posts for three years, after which alternative funding is required, for example from the health authority. The study was conducted over eighteen months and funded by CRMF.

Nursing education has been and continues to be subject to major reform. The basis and system of training has altered radically with the introduction of Project 2000 (UKCC, 1986). Post-Registration Education and Practice (PREP) proposes that continuing education should be mandatory (UKCC, 1990). The recommendations in both Project 2000 and PREP assume that nurse education will be strongly linked with the Higher Education sector. These changes impact on the role of nurse teachers. There are also implications in relation to the preparation of nurse teachers for their role.

In 1989 the Department of Health proposed that by 1995 all newly appointed nurse teachers should be graduates (DoH, 1989). In addition, the English National Board (ENB) commented that, 'Specialisation amongst nurse teachers should be encouraged; tutor students should have the opportunity to study a specialist clinical subject in depth' (ENB, 1989). There is an awareness that the days of the generic teacher are over; no one teacher can possibly have the depth of knowledge required across all subjects (Kenworthy, 1985; Wood, 1987; Gallego and Walter, 1991;

Burke, 1993). Moreover, there is a recognition that specialisms and specialist teachers need to be rooted in practice. Gallego and Walter (1991) argue that specialisms 'need to be examined and developed in the context of practice since specialist knowledge cannot survive in a theoretical vacuum' (p95). Thus the MNT post is an example of the moves within nurse education towards having specialist posts which encompass both the academic and clinical aspects of nursing.

Methods

A qualitative approach was used, as it is well suited to exploring persons' experiences and interactional relationships (Strauss and Corbin, 1990). Qualitative methods can be used to uncover and understand what lies behind things, and to provide new angles on seemingly well-known areas (Strauss and Corbin, 1990).

Data collection was by means of semi-structured, open-ended interviews which were tape-recorded and transcribed verbatim. An aide-mémoire was used with an emphasis on follow-up questions, areas were explored rather than specific questions asked. The topics discussed included tutors' career history, who, what and where they taught, what they perceived their role to be, their working relationships, and the impact on their role of changes in nurse education and the delivery of health care. CRMF supplied a list of all MNTs in England and Wales funded either currently or in the past, which totalled forty-five. (There are only three male MNTs and to protect their identity the female pronoun will be used throughout.) The potential respondents were contacted by telephone or letter, followed by a phone call, the purpose of the study was explained, confidentiality assured (all names of people or places are pseudonyms, borrowed or adapted from *Nicholas Nickleby* by Charles Dickens) and permission to tape-record the interview obtained. All those approached were willing to participate and were very cooperative, fitting the interview into their busy schedules. Many of the MNTs expressed a keen interest in the study and this is reflected in the rich and full accounts they gave.

MNTs do not operate in isolation; they work within a collegial network and many straddle two very different work settings. In order to place MNTs into the broader context and to examine the posts in more depth, two case studies were conducted. The role sets of two MNTs (figures 3.1 and 3.2) were interviewed about their perceptions of the MNT role, the impact of the educational and health reforms on the institution and on the role of the MNT.

Sample

The MNT interviews were conducted in three stages, the starting point being two experienced tutors recommended by CRMF. In addition to being interviewed they commented on the aide-mémoire and through their extensive knowledge of the

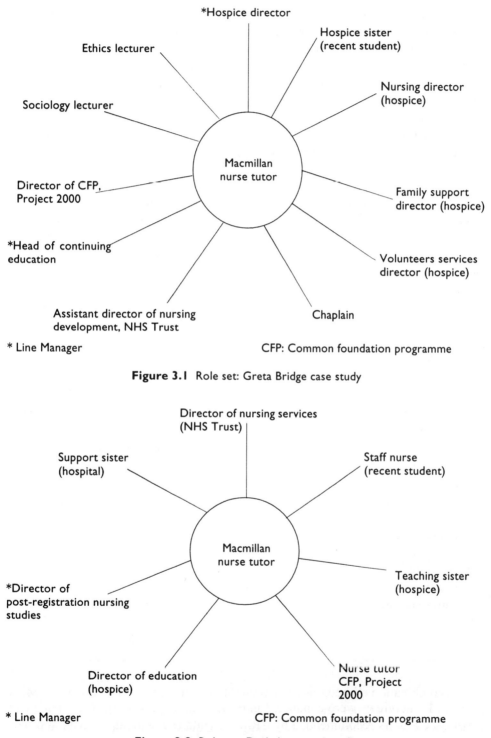

Figure 3.1 Role set: Greta Bridge case study

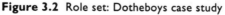

Figure 3.2 Role set: Dotheboys case study

MNT network suggested possible subjects. After 11 interviews and with eight transcripts available, preliminary analysis was conducted using Straussian coding techniques. Coding is a process of breaking down, examining, comparing and conceptualising and categorising the data (Strauss and Corbin, 1990). This was done to refine the focus of the study by identification of key categories and concepts. A further eleven interviews were conducted, the sample being driven by the data until theoretical saturation was achieved. This occurred when no new or relevant data seemed to emerge, categories had been well developed and relationships between categories were established (Strauss and Corbin, 1990). (See tables 3.1 and 3.2).

Table 3.1 The MNT sample by specialty and grant status

	Current CRMF grant	Post–CRMF grant	Total
Palliative care	7	9	16
Cancer care	2	3	5
Palliative and cancer care	1	0	1
Total	10	12	22

Table 3.2 The MNT sample by specialty and appointment

	Joint appt	College based	Clinically based	Total
Palliative care	12	2	2	16
Cancer care	0	4	1	5
Palliative and cancer care	0	1	0	1
Total	12	7	3	22

The combination of methods used in this study allowed the diversity of the MNT posts to be mapped out and then considered in depth. The data from the MNT interviews informed the case studies, suggesting questions to ask and whom to ask.

The case studies allowed other voices to be heard, so that alternative perspectives of the MNT role were obtained. Thus, the many facets of the role which emerged from the MNT interviews were explored in the context in which the MNT has to operate.

A small-scale study focusing on a specific group of tutors has its limitations. Although respondents were asked to look back and to the future, this study really represents a 'snapshot'. A longitudinal study would allow changes over time to be mapped out. This study attempts to portray the experiences of a particular group of tutors and as such cannot make claims about the experience of other groups of nurse tutors. The focus of this paper will be around issues of context and culture which emerged as major themes in this study. The organisational culture of hospices and Colleges will be mapped out in order to explore the contrasts and the conflicts and to consider the impact of the market-led reforms.

Organisational Culture: Contrasts and Conflicts

MNTs holding joint appointments, particularly between a hospice and a College of Nursing, often highlight the differences between the two. As one tutor said: 'How can one have allegiance to two organisations who have very, very different styles and approaches? I can't feel equal allegiance to both' (N. Crummles, MNT). This raises questions not just about the difficulties of having two 'masters' but also the idea that organisations embody different sets of values and beliefs, that they have distinct cultures.

The Hospice 'Culture'

With one or two exceptions, the working environment provided by hospices is described in glowing terms. In general, hospices are described as places where MNTs feel valued, trusted and supported in their work.

Hospices are small, often charitable organisations; their conception and establishment is usually the result of a concerted campaign by a group of committed local people, both professional and non-professional. Within hospices there appears to be a strong sense of 'community', of belonging to and being responsible to the community. As a director of a hospice commented: 'We are very much a community project and of course the people are all part of the community, so it's their hospice and that gives us a bonus.' She continued, 'We are not, as it were, an independent organisation, we are the community's organisation' (T. Linkinwater, hospice director). A hospice colleague described an MNT:

'She's not a sort of a pure educationalist in academic terms . . . she's very much a community educationalist too . . . and I think that's great, I really do, and I think . . . we can see how she's networking out there amongst our health colleagues, but also the community as well, so I see her as a great facilitator of education and learning . . . about palliative care . . . on many many different levels.'

(L. Cheeryble, social worker)

Lucy Cheeryble suggested that as the hospice was part of the community this gave the MNT 'licence' to go out into the wide world. Another link with the community is provided by the numerous volunteers who work at hospices, providing a wide range of skills from gardening to bereavement counselling. These volunteers act as 'ambassadors' for hospices as they return to their homes and workplaces. Most hospices have education and training for volunteers with the MNTs contributing to these programmes.

Services that hospices provide develop over time, maybe beginning with inpatient and domiciliary services, then developing daycare facilities. Once the services and staff have 'matured', education programmes can be developed: 'One aspect about the hospice is it has a very very heavy commitment to education. Having established as it were a patient care system, its future, right from the beginning, was geared towards education as well' (T. Linkinwater, hospice director). Hospices recognise that they provide direct care for a privileged few and thus the aim of their educational programme is to take the principles of palliative care to all arenas of care. As one MNT commented: 'Nobody here that I know in the hospice thinks that palliative care can only be done in a hospice.' Moreover there is a 'very very clear philosophy that you can improve care in a big way through education' (N. Crummles, MNT). Hospices strive to share their skills with a diverse group, from schoolchildren to health care professionals, and use their standing in the community to establish information networks.

MNTs often say that they feel valued and trusted by their hospice colleagues: 'It's easier to have some freedom to work here [hospice] – I feel I'm allowed to do what I'm good at' (N. Crummles, MNT). Within hospices MNTs are generally regarded as senior members of staff. In the Greta Bridge case study the MNT was part of the senior staff team along with the medical director, nursing director, administrator, social worker, fundraiser, volunteer coordinator and chaplain who formed the day-to-day management team and reported to the hospice director. The director commented that in the MNT, 'I am making a very senior appointment, and I expect in making that appointment to appoint someone who is able to manage themselves, and use their own professional discretion as to what they're doing' (T. Linkinwater, hospice director). Within the hospice MNTs are thus 'fairly autonomous'; a contrast is often drawn with their position in the college of nursing where they are called to account much more. As Ninetta Crummles, quoted above, commented, 'There aren't the boundaries that there are within the big organisation in the college.'

Hospices are described as providing a nurturing environment where support is 'a way of life'. The support networks are informal; there is a lot of problem-sharing and awareness of each other. 'There's a lot of looking out for each other in a place like this . . . you know if you see someone's upset . . . if I see someone's upset . . . if appropriate, I would offer help – and people do that for me' (N. Crummles, MNT). Within joint appointments senior hospice staff are described as more understanding about the difficulties of having two masters and the potential for an evergrowing workload. An MNT commented that while the college 'want an extra pound of flesh all the time' (M. Mantalini, MNT), the hospice acknowledged the need for boundaries.

MNTs recognise that hospices, as they are separate from mainstream health care and are comfortable places to work in, are in danger of becoming insular and isolated: 'The risk of professional isolation in what is a registered nursing home, effectively, could be great' (P. Lillyvick, MNT). Indeed, MNTs and their hospice colleagues regard MNTs as an important link with the 'outside' world of education and the NHS. There is an awareness that in order to be a centre of excellence staff must keep their skills and knowledge up to date, and moreover that it is to a large extent the responsibility of the hospice to support the education of their staff:

'I think if we are setting ourselves up as a centre of excellence then we need to definitely say okay, we're going to put our . . . we've said that, we're going to put our money where our mouth is basically, and I think that's very important, that we have a responsibility . . . that we can't bring people in, attract them by being a centre of excellence, and then they regress by being here, that's very important.'

(M. Bray, nursing director, hospice)

She goes on:

'Well, I feel that must have an influence on how they work. If the culture of the organisation is about progression and learning and all of that and communicating and enabling . . . which I hope it's what it's about and not, as you say, coming and do that little bit, and it's about working together as a team to develop in the future of palliative care . . . I think that can only benefit in the future people, 'cos they're going to go on and wherever they go they're gonna be good practitioners, and I think there is a responsibility on that.'

This view of education as a long-term process which involves personal development, benefiting the community as a whole not just the institution and requiring investment by the employer, is very much a 'global' view of education. Such a notion is underpinned with a sense of collective responsibility for education and a belief that education can in practical terms improve the care that the dying receive.

In general, hospices are described by MNTs as 'good' places to work in, but there are exceptions. Several MNTs have faced resistance, particularly when trying to get staff to take a more active role in their own learning and professional development. These tutors feel that their role is not understood and there is a resistance to innovation and change. It is the 'matrons' who are regarded as the stumbling blocks, being described as controlling and prescriptive. So that although education may be encouraged, this is only done within the framework endorsed by the matron. MNTs who strive to introduce fresh ideas can find obstacles put in their way, such as staff not being released from their clinical duties. Within the culture of the hospice, the questioning, reflective, self-directed approach, where individuals take on more responsibility for their own learning, appears to constitute a threat.

Also in a small unit, where a lot of staff, including the senior people, have been in post for many years, the prospect of an 'outsider' introducing change can be very threatening. One MNT who had been a Sister in the hospice found that when she took on the label of 'tutor' barriers were created and she was treated as an 'outsider', for example being excluded from social gatherings. So that while in general hospices are supportive, nurturing and keen to develop palliative care both within and beyond the hospice, some are insular and defensive. It may be that tutors as 'outsiders' are deemed to constitute a threat to the stability of the organisation, by introducing new ideas, opening the minds of the staff and the doors of the hospice.

The Educational Institution 'Culture'

In recent years, Colleges of Nursing have undergone major changes and more are in the pipeline. Formerly, Colleges of Nursing were relatively small, monotechnic institutes, with few if any links with other Colleges or other forms of education. These Colleges were managed by nurses, funded from a range of sources and were fairly autonomous.

The introduction of Project 2000, with the need to broaden the academic base and the introduction of market philosophies to health care and education, has led to amalgamations of colleges and the formation of links with Higher Education. The result has been large Colleges, perhaps straddling several counties and spread out on numerous sites. This period of change has meant early retirement for some, new jobs for others, changing working practices and relationships for everyone and above all uncertainty.

Changing Values and Priorities

The working environment provided by the College is described by the MNTs in primarily negative terms. Both the physical working conditions and the culture attract criticism. Several MNTs said they based themselves at the hospice rather than the College because the accommodation on offer was superior. This is how one MNT described the College:

'They are bursting at the seams as far as accommodation goes. They've got some wonderful people in there, they've got business managers and resource managers and this that and the other managers, and there is no room for tutors there.'

She continued:

'I've got sort of a quarter of a shared office, there's about five other people come in and out, it's like Piccadilly Circus . . . no room for my books, and you really can't work . . . there's one phone between five, it's just not feasible . . . you really can't work.'

(M. Price, MNT)

She contrasts this to the hospice, 'where I can have an office, with my books, filing cabinets and all the rest of it.' Such seemingly mundane issues as space occupation can reflect the values of the institution and in particular who is valued. Educationalists feel they have been displaced by managers who are valued highly within the current political climate.

In addition, several MNTs express concern that they and the courses they devise are being judged not for their educational worth but their financial worth. For one tutor who had just had a diploma validated by both the ENB and a university, her worry was: 'It may well be that I feel that I've created something that's worthwhile, but if the values that I have don't convert into financial returns, it may be judged to be of no value,' and in her words: 'You will be dispensed with' (J. Wititterly, MNT). MNTs seem to regard the period of the CRMF grant as the time in which they have to prove themselves as 'almost indispensable'. There is an awareness amongst the MNTs that to survive within the educational marketplace the college will place greater emphasis on income generation:

'I think I have more altruistic reasoning and whilst it's important to generate some money that should not be the sole reason for existence. But there is a growing recognition from many senior educationalists . . . that the death and dying arena is an area where a lot of money can be made, and I do not want pressure to make money above all else.'

(P. Lillyvick, MNT)

There appears to be shifting of values away from what might be termed professional educational to market values. Meek (1988) maintains that several cultures can coexist within an organisation, and in one of the case studies a colleague of the MNT felt that what had emerged was 'at least two identifiable cultures'.

She continued:

> 'There's one which I call the professional educational culture, where the emphasis is very very much upon education and professional values, and I think a lot of my nursing colleagues would echo what I've said about the market economy and the rest. And then there's a managerial culture, with all the managerial rhetoric that goes with this, and . . . the market rhetoric and so on and so forth, of selling . . . creating new products for the market, and marketing them, selling these things.'

> (F. Verisopht, sociology lecturer)

This shift of values is for many partial and as the above quotes indicate there is a degree of resistance from educationalists. It is perhaps, as Feldman (1986) argues, more difficult to produce a homogeneous culture than the prescriptive texts, such as *In Search of Excellence* (Peters and Waterman, 1982), suggest.

Nevertheless, there appears to be some value confusion, with MNTs either unsure as to what criteria were being used to assess educational courses or uncomfortable with the criteria, for example the 'money-making' potential of a course. Several MNTs were fundamentally opposed to the market model; as one said: 'That doesn't fit in with my philosophy of overall palliative care, in providing as wide a possibility without overlapping and competing, so I don't like that at all' (A. Browdie, MNT). The values of the market appears to have been absorbed much more by those in managerial positions, or perhaps they have been appointed to those posts because of the values they hold. One educational manager, who spoke the language of the market, said:

> 'The organisation as a whole needs to survive as a corporate entity, so we have a mission statement, we know where we want to go, it's a long-term goal, but we also know that the way of getting there, we need to reach certain milestones, so we have immediate, intermediate and long-term objectives . . . I think the current market highlights certain values, and I think they are congruent with the core values of nursing . . . like . . . those values are student-centred learning, the same as patient-centred care, accountability again is out there, the emphasis on quality . . . again I think all these are core values with nursing and with care so I don't have a problem with that . . . Personally I do not see that the current market ethos is a constraint, I think it gives tremendous scope, to take the initiative and to run with it.'

> (P. Sliderskew, head of continuing education)

Such views are at odds with those of many MNTs who feel that market values are antithetical to the holistic model of care that underpins palliative care.

Views and Beliefs about Education

Colleges as providers of education within the marketplace have to be responsive to the requests of the purchasers of education. Service managers argue that education needs to be more flexible: 'It tends to be 9 to 5, Monday to Friday and the library is the same. Most people work during those hours – they can't get there' (M. Bray, nursing director, hospice). Moreover the cost of replacing staff who have been released for educational courses is inhibiting in a health service dominated by budgetary considerations. One NHS trust manager described herself as 'the voice of the directorate' whose role was to ensure that 'they had the right training courses at the right times of year and we've also just developed a quality specification with the college, saying we don't want courses running during the summer weeks, during Christmas, whatever. So we feel more in control . . . We're looking at the courses being delivered in afternoon sessions, as opposed to two-week blocks, whole days, things like that' (L. Bravassa, assistant director nursing development, NHS trust). Thus the relationship between education and service is changing, with colleges reorganising courses at the behest of service and having to demonstrate the effectiveness of the education they provide: 'How do the practitioners come out different at the end, and if they don't come out different then what's the point of sending people?' (L. Bravassa, assistant director nursing development, NHS trust). Furthermore, in considering a practitioner's request for funding and/or study leave, Lily Bravassa maintains:

'The needs of the service have to be the focus . . . whilst professional development fits into that, the individual has to take second place to the needs of service, so it would be the service that would dictate to a large extent the availability of courses.'

Lily Bravassa suggests the culture of the trust she works in is changing, with people being much more critical and analytical of the educational courses that staff attend. Educational courses are now subject to repeated evaluation, with aims and objectives being stated, competencies set, so that 'visible outcomes' can be measured and demonstrated. For Lily Bravassa and Peg Sliderskew such an approach is the way forward, whilst others, including some MNTs, regard it as too mechanistic, focusing on technical skills, short-term outcomes and the needs of the institution, negating certain aspects of education – for instance personal development. Thus, there is a tension between the institutional view of education held by some managers and the global view of education held by many educationalists. The global view of education sits uneasily within the prevalent culture of measurement and audit:

'Sometimes it's actually very very difficult to justify what we are doing in terms of a narrow notion of relevance. I mean one could perhaps argue that the broad liberal education has its relevance, and does translate into better practice, but it's very very difficult to measure this, or to quantify it, or to identify in what precise way this occurs. I'm personally sure it does happen, but it's much more difficult to advance that particular argument.'

She continued:

'The old notion of holistic care and all the rest of it is very very nebulous, it's much more easy to talk about task performance, isn't it, to actually work along a model where you can actually quantify tasks that have to be carried out in relation to patient care, than issues of communication skills and talking to patients, and being alive to the emotional world of patients, and the social circumstances of patients . . . and how this may impinge upon their treatment. Again very very difficult things to quantify.'

(F. Verisopht, sociology lecturer)

Such concerns are echoed by MNTs who fear that the emphasis on training and information could have a detrimental effect on palliative care:

'I'm also concerned that because of the difficulties that people have with death and dying, they're not measurable . . . people can see if somebody's not given a bed bath, people can see if injections aren't getting done, but if people are not communicating very well there's all sorts of problems . . . It takes a brave patient to complain . . . and therefore I think it could become low priority with some managers.'

(K. Nickleby, MNT)

Peg Sliderskew (head of continuing education) dismisses the idea that some aspects of education and patient care are unquantifiable as 'myth' perpetuated by teachers and practitioners.

The market values that underpin the institutional/managerial view of education are clearly expressed in relation to the question: who should pay for post-registration education? In the case studies both the managers responsible for post-basic education provided similar responses:

'Personally I believe that the individual has responsibility for their personal development . . . so I believe the individual has to make an investment into themselves, they have to contribute to their personal development, but I also feel that from an organisation perspective, I feel that in order for the organisation to gain from its workforce they have to invest in their workforce.'

(P. Sliderskew, head of continuing education)

'If I can say from a personal perspective, and I think it's something that I feel quite strongly about, and maybe it is the wrong area to feel strongly about, but I do feel that if we are to be seen as a profession, we personally should be paying for those courses, and that is a totally personal view.'

(A. Snevellicci, director of post-basic education)

The notion of individualism is further underscored by the requirement of many trusts that staff 'repay' any investment made, by working for a year and in some cases two years – if staff leave within that time they have to repay the costs of the course. Such ideas contrast strongly with those held by many of the teachers and practitioners within the case studies:

'I think in an ideal world it would be best if there were some form of quite independent form of funding, divorced from the service side, making staff less dependent upon the favours of service, and the funding from central funding body, but . . . that sounds very very utopian today, but that I think is the ideal requirement.'

(F. Verisopht, sociology lecturer)

'Well, I always feel strongly that an employer should fund education and training, that ought to be a commitment that all employers undertake if they're going to employ people, because it helps people do their job and develop . . . so I think fundamentally employers should undertake it.'

(L. Cheeryble, social worker, hospice)

Lucy Cheeryble lamented the dwindling amount of money allocated for education:

'Because actually the resource at the end of the day is the people who are doing the jobs . . . and if we don't invest in their training and education, what's the point in having wonderful stocks of bandages and medication if people aren't quite sure what they are doing?'

The 'Sausage Machine': the New Generation of Colleges of Nursing

For many MNTs used to working in small Colleges where everyone knew each other, the new generation of Colleges strikes them as huge and impersonal. For those MNTs in joint appointments with hospices the contrast is often sharper still; at the hospice they are part of a small team who all know each other, while at the college, 'they are all sorts of faces floating around and nobody knows who they are – you don't know whether they're the secretary, a cleaner or the new vice principal' (M. Price, MNT). Several MNTs conjure up Kafkaesque images of individuals beavering behind firmly closed doors, never venturing out during the working day, thus quite oblivious of each other's existence, as one MNT commented: 'In spite of all my efforts, I am quite sure that there are some people in the college who actually don't know that there's a Macmillan tutor on the staff . . . after three years' (M. Price, MNT).

One MNT described the College as fostering a 'culture of neglect', another that the atmosphere was not 'congenial', with several MNTs commenting that they felt there was no one within the College that they could approach for support. For another who had to resubmit her MPhil, 'I was devastated to find I hadn't passed, and the support I got over here [hospice] was tremendous, and over in the college the majority of people just sort of passed it off, oh shame, end of story' (N. Crummles, MNT). For one MNT the college was a 'sausage machine' designed to churn out more and more students, with little regard for the social wellbeing of students or staff. This sense of isolation and demoralisation is deepened by the distant managerialism which now dominates in college administration. Many MNTs speak of numerous appointments broken by managers:

> 'Well, she's verbally willing, but we've had many appointments which she had to cancel at the last minute . . . because she has a huge workload and commitment . . . so . . . it isn't one of her priorities, particularly with all the amalgamations and the push for courses to be validated with the university.'
>
> (A. Browdie, MNT)

One MNT, an experienced teacher, describes a change from the days when the Principal's door was always open, 'literally not just a metaphorically open door, but she left her door standing open, so you didn't feel you even had to knock, it was that sort of openness' (M. Price, MNT), to nowadays with the 'new leadership' where appointments are frequently broken and for her 'that says a lot about who is valued.' Furthermore, MNTs are frequently left uninformed about the funding arrangements at the end of the CRMF grant, as one MNT commented: 'I was told . . . in retrospect actually your salary was paid out of a different fund, as from last month . . . that's how I eventually knew' (A. Browdie, MNT).

The sustained, top-down pressure for change is reflected in the atmosphere of Colleges which is described in terms of 'madness' by several MNTs: 'There is so much going on . . . there is a mad rush . . . you've got to get your link with higher education tied up, there is meeting after endless meeting,' for this MNT it was 'mad, mad, chaos', another referred to an 'undercurrent of hysteria'. The pace and number of changes leave MNTs and their colleagues feeling weary and demoralised, as one MNT explained:

> 'I think it is difficult, I mean change is important and change is necessary but I think we seem to be in a total round of change all the time now, and the dust doesn't get time to settle and then something else occurs and there's no way of evaluating what's going on and seeing whether it's actually working or if it isn't because it's changed.'
>
> (S. La Creevy, MNT)

For another: 'I think I'm like that woman in Stevie Smith's "Not waving but drowning" . . . I think most of the time I keep my head above water' (M. Mantalini, MNT). MNTs are having to take on new roles and acquire new skills, which they have not been trained for and in some cases do not relish:

> 'I think I'm in a sort of position that a lot of nurses are in where . . . your background . . . training . . . didn't lead you to believe that writing or publishing was something you did really . . . if that makes sense . . . and since I've come into education it's more expected.'
>
> (F. Squeers, MNT)

For another, in relation to the requirement to 'sell' education: 'I just wonder what I am sometimes. I'm feeling quite . . . sort of a cross between a con-man and something else . . . income generation is something that is really alien, isn't it?' (J. Wititterly, MNT). Moreover, 'It's something that has been thrust onto people which people are not used to doing' (S. La Creevy, MNT). MNTs, like all nurse tutors, are striving to find a place within academia at a time when higher education is undergoing change; the market is as new and unsettling for Higher Education lecturers as it is for nurse tutors.

Discussion

The working environment of MNTs is in a state of flux, partly as a result of government policy and partly because of moves within nursing to strengthen the profession. The criteria by which all educationalists are judged are being reformulated, with the new touchstones being 'economy', 'efficiency' and 'effectiveness'. For MNTs in joint appointments the contrast between the two organisations is often stark. This is not to say that hospices are not touched by market forces; while they may not be, as a hospice director put it, 'sophisticatedly money-orientated', they are 'having to be increasingly financially sophisticated' (T. Linkinwater, hospice director). The difference seems to be in the underlying values which set the agenda and priorities of each institution. Some MNTs describe a 'growing apart', with Colleges moving further down the market road whilst hospices continue to aim to improve palliative care services by creating opportunities for their expertise to be shared with all those concerned with the care of the dying.

Within Colleges and service providers a narrow, institutional and technical skill-orientated view of education is challenging the broader, global view of education which acknowledges the long-term and seemingly intangible benefits of education for the individual and the community. Many educationalists, MNTs amongst them, are striving to uphold this global view of education and the associated professional educational culture in what can be viewed as a war of attrition between the professions and the managers. Education can play a pivotal role in this resistance, but this is partly dependent on education resisting the calls of service managers to tailor courses entirely to the 'needs' of service; that is, readily quantified skills.

This is not to say that MNTs reject the market-led reforms out of hand – indeed they have been able to exploit them to their advantage, for instance by increasing access to palliative care education through flexible learning packages. Nonetheless, many MNTs express concern about health care and educational systems being dominated by market philosophies. As Bartlett and Le Grand (1993) argue, many people working in public services find it difficult to shift from considering the welfare of their users to the financial health of their provider unit.

The agreements for the funding and management of MNT posts have had an air of informality. Within this study there is an acknowledgement that such informal arrangements are not appropriate to the educational marketplace. Indeed, the current contract culture can provide safeguards not only for the MNT's job but for CRMF's investment. A written contract with the duties and responsibilities of all concerned parties agreed and laid out in full could have prevented many of the recent disputes. Particular attention needs to be paid to the financial arrangements not just in relation to funding the post but to the destiny of any income generated. Moreover, it needs to be clear that income generation should be incidental to the MNT's primary educational role.

During this period of intense change MNTs require support. Within this study Colleges of Nursing do not appear adequately to facilitate or support the professional development of nurse tutors. This support needs to be on several levels, including training and an acknowledgement of the time required to fulfil these new roles. Moreover, MNTs must feel they are valued members of the College. This is an area which needs to be addressed if MNTs are going to take on the multi-faceted role envisaged in the new order; as researcher, practitioner and teacher.

References

Bartlett W and Le Grand J (1993) The Theory of Quasi-Markets. In: Le Grand J and Bartlett W (eds) *Quasi-Markets and Social Policy*. London: Macmillan.

Burke L (1993) The future of the specialist nurse teacher: Two different models explored. *Nurse Education Today* 13:40–6.

DoH (1989) *Education and Training: Working Paper 10*. London: HMSO.

ENB (1989) *Preparation of Teachers, Practitioners/Teachers, Mentors and Supervisors in the Context of Project 2000*. London: English National Board for Nursing, Midwifery and Health Visiting.

Feldman SP (1986) Management in context: An essay on the relevance of culture to the understanding of organizational change. *Journal of Management Studies* 23(6):587–607.

Gallego A and Walter P (1991) Preparation of health care teachers for the future. *Nurse Education Today* 11:94–9.

Kenworthy N (1985) Specialist roles for nurse teachers. *Nurse Education Today* 5:37–40.

Meek VL (1988) Organizational culture: Origins and weaknesses. *Organization Studies* **9**(4):453–73.

Peters T and Waterman RH (1982) *In Search of Excellence.* New York: Harper and Row.

Strauss A and Corbin J (1990) *Basics of Qualitative Research: Grounded Theory and Procedures and Techniques.* Newbury Park, California: Sage.

UKCC (1986) *Project 2000: A New Preparation for Practice.* London: United Kingdom Central Council for Nursing, Midwifery and Health Visiting.

UKCC (1990) *The Report of the Post-registration and Practice Project.* London: United Kingdom Central Council for Nursing, Midwifery and Health Visiting.

Wood V (1987) The nurse instructor and the teaching climate. *Nurse Education Today* **7**:228–34.

Chapter 4
Creating a 'Seamless Web of Care' – The Work of Paediatric Oncology Outreach Nurse Specialists

Sarah Bignold, Alan Cribb
and Stephen J. Ball

This chapter is based upon a research project conducted at King's College London in 1992 and 1993. In the light of the brief outlined by the funding agencies, Cancer Relief Macmillan Fund and the Department of Health, the aim of our research was to reach an understanding of the needs and experiences of families with children with cancer and how paediatric oncology outreach nurse specialists (POONSs) help to meet these needs. In this chapter we present a brief outline of the research, the impact that childhood cancer has on families and how POONSs help to create a 'seamless web of care' for families. We then consider three sets of issues that reflect the challenging nature of the POONS role. In the concluding section we summarise the key elements that underpin the supportive role of POONSs.

Background

Since the late 1960s the treatment of childhood cancer has improved dramatically so that now 60–70 per cent of children will survive the disease. At the same time treatment has tended to become more aggressive and to take place over longer periods of time, often over two years or more. These changes have coincided with a growing body of research that shows the deleterious effects of prolonged hospitalisation on young children, as a result, for example, of disruption to their daily lives and anxiety due to separation from their family and home (Prugh *et al*, 1953; Bowlby, 1969; Robertson, 1970). This has led to a new emphasis upon caring for children in their own homes and avoiding hospitalisation wherever possible. In a recent study While (1992) has indicated that home care enhances the family's sense of normality and that parents believe this is conducive to their child's well-being.

These changed patterns of care mean that children undergoing treatment for cancer now spend much longer periods of time in their own homes. Although home care is clearly valued it can, paradoxically, give rise to new problems. The rarity of childhood cancer means that professional carers in the community are unlikely to have had much, if any, previous experience of caring for such children. They are therefore ill-equipped to deal with their needs and this can create a sense of insecurity and vulnerability for families. It was indeed this sense of vulnerability that led to the inception of the first POONS posts in the mid 1980s, often as a result of the fund-raising activities of parents. The following quotations from the data illustrate this point.

'It was originally set up in March 1989 . . . as a result of the parents . . . because this is the regional centre for quite a wide area, and parents were coming and then going back home. And they identified a need . . . that they felt really isolated when they went back home.'

(S. Hearns, POONS)

'We all felt, through personal experience . . . that there was this great divide between the hospital, you know, where you went with your child, and everybody knew what you were talking about and there was great expertise . . . and there was the community where nobody knew anything, and you felt very vulnerable and alone, and so I mean . . . it has always been an idea that we really wanted to have a nurse . . . who was actually based in the hospital, but could also cross both barriers and come out into the community and see the children at home. So you know, you've got a sort of liaison both ways . . . and you help the families when they were most vulnerable, at home . . . especially with terminal care . . . and that's what we've done.'

(D. Smith, Parent and Charity Trustee)

Since the mid 1980s there has been a rapid growth of POONS posts so that there are now about 40 POONSs throughout the country. The nurses are funded by charities such as Cancer Relief Macmillan Fund and the Cancer and Leukaemia in Childhood Trust or by the NHS. The POONSs are paediatric-trained nurses; most have had experience in paediatric oncology prior to taking up their posts, some have had previous experience in community nursing and a few have had previous experience in both paediatric oncology and community nursing. The POONSs are based in hospital and predominantly at the specialist paediatric oncology centres. The nurses form a strong professional network, meeting together four times a year at the Royal College of Nursing, attending conferences together and maintaining contact by telephone. Despite the rapid growth of the POONSs posts their services have never been formally evaluated. It was for these reasons that we were asked by

Cancer Relief Macmillan Fund (one of the major funders of the posts) and the Department of Health to conduct an independent review of their work. Such a review was deemed necessary before any further expansion of the posts and to inform future policy.

About the Research

Our work was conducted according to the canons of qualitative research which allowed us to be open, holistic and fairly exhaustive in relation to the major issues identified within the research. As Gilgun (1992) has said, 'the processes of qualitative research include ways of conceptualising, collecting, analysing and interpreting data' (p24). The primary technique for data collection was the unstructured interview based upon the use of an aide-mémoire of issues and topics to be discussed. All interviews were tape-recorded and professionally transcribed. The analysis of these transcripts and the guiding principles of the research were based upon the constant comparative method, as developed by Glaser and Strauss (1967). That is to say, the main emphasis was upon discovery, and analysis was sequential – it was guided by and guided data collection. Key categories and their properties were identified in the data and 'saturated' – that is, checked and re-checked against further data, elaborated and reformulated. This was achieved both by the intensive coding of transcripts and by the use of analytic insights derived from the coding to organise and focus further data collection.

Eighty-six interviews were conducted in the course of the research. Thirty-five interviews were carried out with parents of children who had or had had cancer; 28 with mothers, one with a father and six with both parents together, making a total of 34 families. The contacts with parents were made in two ways, that is either through self-help group organisers, or via nurses at two of the specialist paediatric oncology centres. At the time of interview 11 children were receiving treatment, 12 had completed treatment, one child was terminally ill and ten children had died. Approximately half of the children were receiving, or had received, all of their treatment at a specialist paediatric oncology centre, and the remaining children were being treated, or had been treated, on a shared care basis; that is, they received at least some of their treatment and related care at a local district hospital under the supervision of the specialist centre. At the time of interview, 12 families had had no access to a POONS, four families had had access to a POONS for part, but not all, of their child's illness trajectory and the remaining 18 families had had continuous access to a POONS from the point of a cancer diagnosis.

Nineteen POONSs were interviewed; 12 were, or had been, funded by Cancer Relief Macmillan Fund and were known as Paediatric Macmillan Nurses; the remainder were funded by other charities or by the NHS. With the exception of two nurses all of the POONSs interviewed were based at specialist paediatric oncology centres and so our findings relate most closely to these nurses. A further 32 interviews were conducted with other professional carers, including paediatric oncology consultants, ward-based nurses, social workers, members of the primary health care team and with POONS managers and advisers.

Families with Children with Cancer

Our interviews with both professional carers and parents show the immense and traumatic impact that a childhood cancer diagnosis has on families. Most parents automatically associate the initial cancer diagnosis with the death of their child. It gives rise to a myriad of extremely painful emotions, including fear, despair, anger and disbelief that this could happen to their child. Furthermore, although there has been a considerable improvement in the treatment of childhood cancer in recent years the actual success of treatment cannot be ascertained for some years after completion of treatment. This means that the experience of childhood cancer is underpinned for families by a chronic uncertainty about their child's survival that lasts not only throughout the rigours of treatment but also into the post-treatment phase. As Koocher and O'Malley (1981) have pointed out, parents are thus faced with the extremely painful task of balancing an awareness of the possibility of death with a realistic hope of their child's survival. The emotional, practical and often financial strain of coping with childhood cancer reverberates around families, affecting not only the child with cancer but the lives and health of all concerned. Marriages are often put under immense strain as partners cope and react differently at different times, siblings often regress or conversely mature beyond their years, some families are resilient, but others are torn apart by the experience.

The treatment for childhood cancer typically takes place over a course of months or years. After a cancer diagnosis is made by the family's GP or local hospital, most children are transferred to a specialist centre where a treatment protocol is devised. An initial block of treatment is given and subsequent treatments and care then continue either at the specialist centre or on a shared-care basis with the family's local hospital. Between treatments children return home. If all possible treatment fails the choice of most families to care for their child at home means that terminal care is based in the community. In the course of the illness trajectory families thus move between two or three different health care settings: the specialist centre, the community and sometimes also their local hospital.

In moving between the different health care settings families move between specialist and non-specialist care; between professional carers who understand the nature and impact of childhood cancer and those whose understandings are limited. Interviews with parents show how they invest their trust in professional carers at the specialist centre, not least because they recognise them as the 'experts' in childhood cancer. The professional carers at the specialist centre understand their child's illness and treatment, they can answer their questions and offer them hope for their child's recovery. In contrast, the rarity of childhood cancer means that professional carers in the primary health care sector, as well as to some extent at local hospitals, tend to lack paediatric oncology experience and knowledge. Many GPs, for example, will see only one case of a childhood cancer in their working lives. Interviews with parents show how this makes it difficult for them to place their trust in non-specialist professional carers and can give rise to a sense of isolation, vulnerability and insecurity when being cared for outside of the specialist centre. These feelings are compounded by the fact that care can easily become poorly coordinated and fragmented as families move between the different health care settings and between different groups of professional carers.

Creating a 'Seamless Web of Care'

Our research indicates that the principal raison d'être of POONSs is to 'bridge the gaps' in care that families can experience as they move between the different health care settings. POONSs thus help to create a 'seamless web of care' for families by being available and accessible throughout the child's illness trajectory – that is, from the point of a cancer diagnosis, through treatment and into the post-treatment or terminal and bereavement phases. By meeting with families at the specialist centre, and sometimes at local hospitals, by talking with them on the telephone and visiting them in their own homes POONSs aim to provide families with a strong support line of specialist knowledge and skills which they embody and which is anchored in the specialist centre. POONSs provide families with information about the child's illness and treatment, give advice, guidance and help in decision making. In the early stages of treatment POONSs are involved in teaching parents the necessary skills to care for their child at home in an effort to reduce the amount of time spent in hospital. There are examples of how POONSs help families to manage the uncertainties in relation to treatment outcomes, through providing encouragement and reassurance and helping them to think in terms of quality of life, particularly when the child has a poor prognosis. Interviews with parents indicate that all of these activities are most valued when they are carried out in the relaxed atmosphere of their own homes rather than in the more clinical atmosphere of the hospital.

At interview parents talked about the POONS as someone who was 'always there for them when needed', as 'knowing exactly what was happening' and as 'being able to answer their questions' and 'relieve their worries'. Parents particularly valued the POONS' befriending, non-judgemental approach and the ease with which they could talk to her. As one mother said, 'She's more like a friend than a nurse. I mean she is a nurse, but she is so sweet . . . well I think she's worth her weight in gold, you can *talk to her* so easily.' Many parents felt that their relationship with the POONS resembled or came close to one of friendship. It challenged their expectation of the normative professional–client relationship based upon formality and hierarchy.

The link that POONSs provide with the specialist centre is also much valued by families and becomes particularly salient in the terminal phase of a child's illness, when parents are caring for their child at home, and after the death of their child. At these times parents who did not have access to a POONS tended to experience a sense of being severed from the specialist centre; from the professional carers with whom they had invested their trust and from other families with children with cancer. One mother, for example, spoke of the considerable distress that she and her husband had experienced, because '[we] really felt that we'd been abandoned by the hospital. You know, you're terminally ill, bye-bye . . . there's nothing we can do'. Another mother said that she felt as if she had had 'her arms chopped off', and another, after the death of her child, expressed anguish over the loss of contact with the specialist centre, which she described as having become 'a big second part of [her] life.'

As well as working directly with families throughout the illness trajectory, POONSs aim to create a 'seamless web of care' by working with other professional carers at local hospitals and in the community. POONSs attend paediatric oncology clinics at local hospitals and work with their staff to increase their knowledge and understanding of paediatric oncology care. They aim to create a link between local hospitals and specialist centres by providing up-to-date information between the two sites on each child's treatment and progress. As the following extract suggests this helps to ensure well coordinated care between the different hospital sites.

'She would tell me what's happened at their last visit to the specialist centre, what's been said, what plans have been made . . . she brings a copy of their particular protocol with their dates on . . . and the most important bit of that is right at the beginning . . . if you've got a new leukaemic for example, her information coming from the specialist centre is weeks ahead of the information I get from the doctors . . . I know what's happening week to week . . . and day to day sometimes . . . and hopefully vice versa, I can keep her informed of patients as they come in.'

(R. Clayton, senior doctor at a local hospital)

The doctor quoted above said that the POONSs had helped him to feel more involved with the specialist centre and provided him with a sense of being 'part of their team'. This sense of team work is also fostered by POONSs when working with professional carers in the community. The support of families within the community health care setting is indeed a major focus of the work of POONSs because it is here that gaps in care can be most painfully experienced by families. In contrast to staff at the specialist centre, families often find themselves with a greater understanding of their child's illness and treatment than members of the primary health care team, and this can undermine the development of a trusting relationship.

'It's horrible when you're talking to somebody that doesn't know as much as what you do and you're not even a nurse, 'cos you learn so much. I mean you learn so much about the Hickman line, and my doctor came out here one night to give Mark some anti-sickness IV, 'cos I never had none at home, and we had to tell him how to put it into the Hickman line.'

(Mrs Baker, mother)

Furthermore, the primary health care team, given their lack of paediatric oncology expertise, may avoid families with children with cancer because they are unsure as to what they can offer in the way of support.

'You are sent home to get on with it. Officially we should have been discharged from that hospital at the end of December and simply left to get on with it, and as far as I could see, there was nobody round here picking up the tab . . . no one. The GP didn't come to see us, nobody from [the health centre] came to see us . . . there was no one, you just go home and you get on with it . . . which is quite staggering . . . And everybody else . . . because he's had cancer . . . therefore it's hands off . . . this is something we can't cope with, so we'll leave them alone, we'll leave them to it, sort of thing . . . which just isn't on, really.'

(Mrs Coulby, mother)

POONSs work, then, to enhance the role of the primary health care team by increasing their understanding of the child's illness and treatment and by giving them insight into the impact that childhood cancer has on families. Although POONSs often serve as key workers to families in the treatment phase of the illness, they keep professional carers in the community informed of the child's progress and where appropriate help to draw them into the family's care. If treatment fails, the choice of most families to care for their terminally ill child at home means that care becomes community-based and there is an increased need for collaboration between POONSs and the primary health care team. POONSs arrange meetings with the primary health care team so that roles can be identified for each professional carer and to ensure that families receive appropriate and well managed care. They share with them their expertise in the palliative care of children and give advice on symptom control. When members of the primary health care team have had little or no previous involvement in the family's care many POONSs conduct joint visits with them to the family's home in order to facilitate a relationship between families and community professional carers and to present a team approach.

Challenges to Creating a 'Seamless Web of Care'

POONSs work, then, directly with families, as well as with other professional carers across the different health care settings, so that as far as possible families receive appropriate support throughout the illness trajectory and experience seamless rather than fragmented care. The POONS role is, however, a particularly challenging one, and this can be illustrated by considering three sets of issues arising from their role. These issues have value for formulating policy concerning nurse management and education. First, in creating a 'seamless web of care' POONSs have to take a flexible approach to their work. Second, POONSs work in and between different health care settings that are defined, 'owned' and managed by different parts of the health care system and this gives rise to the possibility of not being recognised, or even of meeting resistance or conflict. Third, a major aspect of their work involves the often difficult and demanding skills of emotional labour. In the remainder of this chapter these three sets of issues will be briefly delineated.

The Need for Flexibility in the Work of POONSs

'And it's really for us to go out and look how we can provide support for that family and meet the individual family's need. I mean again, some families need a lot of support, they want that, they need it, and it's important for them. But some families it's equally important for them to go through this period in their life as a family unit. I think the important thing is they need to know that there are people around for them when they need them.

(B. Mitchell, POONS)

As this extract shows, POONSs have to be sensitive to the individual needs of families. In particular they make themselves available and accessible to families and are 'responsive to demands'. This means avoiding standardised packages of care where routine visits are carried out at certain stages along the illness trajectory. The needs of families can also vary across time and POONSs have to be prepared to increase support when necessary and sometimes to change their plans at short notice.

'We are very flexible, and as I say once a child is terminally ill, palliative care is our number one priority . . . they can bleep us and we'll drop anything. I mean we will go out at any time . . . so if you've got teaching, other home visits arranged, or meetings with people, I mean we just cancel them . . .'

(C. Goff, POONS)

For the most part, this need for flexibility was understood by POONS' managers. When it wasn't, however, POONSs could experience difficulties in executing their role.

'It was this constant querying of everything I did . . . you know . . . do you really think that mother needs like a bereavement visit . . . you're going once a week, is that not too much, do you not think you should lengthen it to four weeks now . . . and this kind of thing . . . to me shows that they didn't understand bereavement . . . that everybody's different, that you couldn't say well look . . . visit all bereaved parents once a week for three weeks . . .'

(A. Pearson, POONS)

The need to avoid standardised packages of care also arises in the *way* in which POONSs increase the families' support in the community health care setting. In the treatment phase POONSs often act as key workers to families, but in the terminal phase they may aim to facilitate community nurses to act in this capacity. The way in which they work with any one family depends upon the needs of individual families, the POONSs' own work pressures and time constraints, the distance that families live from the specialist centre and the resources in the community – for example, whether or not families have access to paediatric community nurses. This calls upon the POONSs' powers of discretion and professional judgement. POONSs cannot be too prescriptive in the way that they work with families and other professional carers; creating a 'seamless web of care' is a creative process in which the individual needs of families have to be recognised, assessed, and matched with the available resources.

Working in and between Different Health Care Settings

POONSs work in and between different health care settings that are defined, 'owned' and managed by different parts of the health care system. POONSs are generally regarded by themselves and others as part of the hospital team (and specifically part of the paediatric oncology team at the specialist centre), and yet they conduct a major part of their role at local hospitals and in the community health care setting where they have no formal rights of entry. Their efforts to establish their role involve *boundary crossing* and this can be perceived as entailing a threat to existing lines of demarcation and roles. Our research highlights how the nature and borders of the different territories can be contested and how POONSs can come across obstacles when attempting to conduct their role in the different health care settings.

'How can we integrate hospital and community, and I suppose as in many other areas a large hospital tends to think that they are at the centre of the world and would like to have outreach services to take over . . . doing all the specialist parts of the community and the community unit feel that hospital is a very small part of the total care of children and should therefore be, if you like, tacked on to the community unit and that debate rages up hill and down dale.'

(E. Davis, Senior Community Nurse)

The successful implementation of the POONSs role means that POONSs have to be prepared to avoid or overcome resistance from other professional carers and to earn their respect. Our research shows that POONSs are remarkably successful at this and that on the whole their relationships with other professional carers are very good. These good relations can be seen to rest upon two foundations. First, POONSs exercise a set of interpersonal skills essential for boundary crossing.

'I try and call and see them informally . . . just to meet and say this is what my job is and I hope you don't mind, because I'm visiting on their territory really and if I can help them with information or anything, feel free to ask, basically.'
(K. Smeddle, POONS)

'I think my way of gaining their trust I guess and support . . . is . . . by going in fairly humbly and saying . . . you know . . . hopefully we'll be able to work together to support this family . . . And if you sort of remain just fairly . . . you know, don't walk in and say . . . I know all about care of dying children and I know what drugs they need, so I'm gonna run the show.'
(T. Jenkins, POONS)

As these extracts show the POONSs' interpersonal skills include tact and diplomacy. Furthermore, because their role is not necessarily or properly understood, POONSs have to be constantly prepared to explain their function and to convince other professional carers of the value of their services. Closely related to this last point is the need for POONSs to demonstrate their willingness to 'work with' rather than simply 'take over' from other professional carers.

Second, because of the 'rarity' of paediatric oncology expertise outside of the specialist centre, POONSs are likely to be perceived as having something valuable to offer in the family's care. They provide a link with the specialist centre for professional carers at local hospitals and in the community and are able to share with them their expertise in paediatric oncology and palliative care of children. In the community health care setting the expertise of POONSs serves to complement the expertise of the primary health care team.

'When I'm working as part of a team, with a family, with the primary health care team . . . then they have got the expertise of working in the community, they know what resources are available to them locally . . . they know how their own primary health care team works in the community and what they want from us, over and above that . . . that they feel they can't give to the families . . . is the expertise in two things . . . one paediatric oncology and if it comes to it, in palliative care of children . . . because it's unlikely that either the GP or the district nurses or health visitors will have had experience with another family.'
(R. Powell, POONS)

Emotional Labour

Throughout the illness trajectory, POONSs share with families and other professional carers their clinical skills and understandings of childhood cancer, but there is also another aspect of their work that is equally pervasive – this is the often difficult and demanding work of emotional labour. Emotional labour has been defined by James (1989) as 'the labour involved in dealing with other people's feelings' (p21). Although emotional labour is part of any professional carer's role it becomes more significant when, as is often the case with POONSs, they are involved with clients undergoing emotional trauma and upheaval over extended periods of time and when they are drawn into the private worlds of their clients. The sense of friendship that often develops between POONSs and families exposes them not only to the practical concerns of families, but also to the families' anxieties, fears, anguish and despair. In supporting families POONSs thus have to help families deal with these difficult feelings. This entails a co-presence, an emotional as well as a physical presence. Although all of the POONSs' work with families is infused with emotional labour they may sometimes visit families for no other reason than to see how they are, to listen to them, to be there for them, and to offer empathy, advice, guidance, encouragement, and reassurance.

As James has pointed out, emotional labour 'demands that the labourer gives personal attention which means they must give something of themselves, not just a formulaic response' (p19). This statement sensitises us to the fact that emotional labour requires the labourer to not only deal with other people's feelings, but also to deal with their own. Our interviews with POONSs certainly highlighted this point.

'You're got to kind of get involved, because you wouldn't be supporting the family particularly well if you were kind of cold towards them. But it's a matter of remaining involved, but trying to keep your feet on hard ground, so that you aren't going to kind of collapse when the family collapse, at the devastation of losing their child . . . so that they've got something to hold on to.'

(A. Harding, POONS)

'I mean it was absolutely tragic that she died, but the good thing was she actually died very peacefully, and she was out of the awful pain which we met as we went through the front door, and I mean actually when she died . . . mum was upset, I cried with mum, because that was actually appropriate, and I was upset . . . but it was just being strong there not to kind of . . . every time I go and see her, you don't kind of . . . you're there to kind of talk through the feelings . . . it's a very difficult thing to explain.'

(A. Harding, POONS)

These extracts show that in supporting families POONSs have to become emotionally involved while at the same time retaining some emotional distance. This means that POONSs have to engage in the self-conscious management of their own feelings. In addition, the second extract shows the difficulty that the POONS had in describing the emotional labour component of her work. Because this type of work is difficult to describe, its challenges and significance in the work of POONSs, and indeed other professional carers, can easily become obscured.

Conclusion

The contrast between the accounts of those parents who had the support of POONSs and those parents who lacked this type of support shows how POONSs are very successful in creating a 'seamless web of care' and how they make a substantial contribution towards reducing and containing at least some of their suffering. From what has been said above the value of the POONS service can be seen to rest upon their ability to combine five key elements in to their role. First, they have the 'rare' expertise in paediatric oncology and the palliative care of children. Second, they provide a strong link with the specialist framework of care for families and other professional carers. Third, they provide families with continuity of care by being available to them throughout the illness trajectory. Fourth, their relationships with families are not merely instrumental but based upon a befriending approach. Fifth, they are able to form effective partnerships with, and provide support to, other professional carers.

Our research suggests that the type of services POONSs provide are not well served by the dominant models of health care evaluation and 'health gain' because they involve complex and diffuse interventions, and they are aimed as much at the process as the output of care. For example, a parent may feel greatly reassured and comforted by the presence of a POONS but this may not be picked up by a scale on psychological morbidity. Narrow models of measurement and evaluation discriminate against certain services so that, as with the work of POONSs, where there is something which is manifestly of value there may be difficulty 'proving' this fact. Those engaged in the management of chronic and life threatening illness need to challenge, rather than 'fit in' with, superficial measures. We believe that qualitative methods, such as those adopted in this study, can be an important means of eliciting and elucidating the value of holistic services.

References

Bowlby J (1969) *Attachment and Loss, 1: Attachment.* Harmondsworth: Penguin.
Gilgun J (1992) Definitions, Methodologies and Methods in Family Research. In: Gilgun J, Daly K and Handel G (eds) *Qualitative Methods in Family Research.* Newbury Park, California: Sage.

Glaser BD and Strauss AL (1967) *The Discovery of Grounded Theory*. New York: Aldine.

James N (1989) Emotional labour: skill and work in the social regulation of feelings. *Sociological Review* **37**(1):15–24.

Koocher GP and O'Malley JE (1981) *The Damocles Syndrome*. New York: McGraw-Hill.

Prugh DG, Staub EM, Sands HH, Kirschbaum RM and Lenihan EA (1953) A study of the emotional reactions of children and families to hospitalisation and illness. *American Journal of Orthopsychiatry* **23**:70–106.

Robertson J (1970) *Young Children in Hospital*. London: Tavistock.

While A (1992) Consumer views of health care: A comparison of hospital and home care. *Child: Care, Health and Development* **18**:107–16.

Section Two

Culture and Society: Implications for Practice

Chapter 5
The Absent Minority: Access and use of Palliative Care Services by Black and Minority Ethnic Groups in Leicester

Hifsa Haroon Iqbal, David Field, Hilda Parker and Zafar Iqbal

'The United Kingdom is now a multicultural, multi-ethnic society and the National Health Service must care for the health of all sectors of the population.'
(Hopkins and Bahl, 1983)

Introduction

This chapter describes a project which examined current service provision and use by the black and minority ethnic groups in Leicester. Little is known about the appropriateness and patterns of uptake of palliative care service provision for the black and minority ethnic groups. The term 'black and minority ethnic group' has been used to refer to people from racial or other minorities who may be discriminated against because of their racial background. There is no single accepted term, nor one which can be seen as being politically correct or incorrect. It should however be recognised that there may be people who do not identify themselves as black or minority but who share a common experience of racism (Anthias, 1992; Cole, 1993).

Although people are aware of the issue, to our knowledge this is the first published examination of palliative care services for the black and minority ethnic groups in the UK. Existing services appear to be underutilised by black and minority ethnic groups. It would appear that access to palliative care services by these groups has been inadequately addressed by individual organisations and purchasing departments.

Background

Leicester is a multiracial, multicultural city with one of the highest overall proportions of black and minority ethnic (BME) populations in the country. Almost 30 per cent of the population in the city of Leicester assessed their ethnicity in categories other than 'white' in the 1991 census (table 5.1) (OPCS, 1991).

Table 5.1 Population configuration for City of Leicester and Leicestershire

	Leicestershire	City of Leicester
Total Persons	867 521	270 493
White	88.9	71.5
Black Caribbean	0.6	1.5
Black African	0.1	0.3
Black Other	0.3	0.6
Indian	8.4	22.3
Pakistani	0.3	1.0
Bangladeshi	0.2	0.4
Chinese	0.2	0.3
Asian/Other	0.4	1.0
Other	0.6	1.1
Total	100%	100%

Source: OPCS (1991)

Research suggests that generally the black and minority ethnic groups in modern Britain have unequal access to services and that their health experiences are worse than for other groups (Burke, 1984; Fernando, 1984; National Association of Health Authorities (NAHA), 1988; Alladin, 1992; Ahmad, 1993; Shaukat et al, 1993). It also seems that generally the black and minority ethnic groups are treated less favourably as a result of racism and the general lack of cultural appreciation which exists among professionals (Parker et al, 1993). One example of this exists in the treatment of psychiatric disorders (Fernando, 1988; Westwood et al, 1989). Other studies have shown that the needs of the individual from the black and minority ethnic groups are being inadequately met (Henley, 1982; Dobson, 1983; Alibhai, 1986).

Professionals dealing with palliative care in Leicestershire from both sides of the purchaser–provider split reported visible evidence that palliative care services were not being used by people from black and minority ethnic groups. These services covered the whole spectrum of care including the hospices, voluntary support agencies and the more specialised hospital-based services. This was a continued concern for health service use in general and was addressed in the local authority's annual report in 1993 (*Health for Leicestershire*, 1993) which concentrated 'on issues which disadvantage some sections of the population in health terms when compared to others'. The study on which this chapter is based was commissioned by Leicestershire Health Authority with the purpose of examining local service provision and of providing a basis for further service development.

Epidemiological Evidence about Cancer in Black and Minority Ethnic Groups

Ethnic origin was first recorded as part of the 1991 National Census, making it possible to have information available on the ethnic composition of Britain (Balarajan and Raleigh, 1991). Ethnic monitoring becomes mandatory for the NHS, initially for inpatients, by April 1995. Although various collections of ethnic data have been made in the past, ethnicity is not yet a factor recorded routinely on NHS databases such as the cancer registry or on death certificates. This makes it difficult to calculate the rates of cancer amongst the black and minority ethnic groups. Despite this lack of accurate data on ethnicity, some published research has attempted to calculate cancer rates by ethnicity. L J Donaldson's paper (1984) identified a higher prevalence of certain cancers amongst Asians such as cancer of the pharynx, oesophagus and mouth. However, he concluded that the prevalence of cancer was lower for Asians when compared with Caucasians. Afro-Caribbeans have been found to have lower cancer rates in the lung, stomach and bowel, but higher rates in the liver and prostate. Overall, the mortality rates from cancer are generally lower for the black and minority ethnic population (Webb, 1982; Cruickshank and Beevers, 1989; Adelstein and Marmot, 1989).

Palliative Care Services

Palliative care has for many years been synonymous with cancer care, though more recently this trend has been redressed, particularly as a result of the Standing Medical/Nursing Advisory Committee Report of 1992 which recommended that palliative care be extended to non-cancer patients. The World Health Organisation defines palliative care as being 'the total care of patients whose disease is not responsive to curative treatments. Control of pain, of other symptoms and of psychological, social and spiritual problems is paramount. The goal of palliative care is achievement of the best possible quality of life for the patient and their families' (Higginson, 1993).

Although palliative care has been extensively studied, there is little published literature on the palliative care needs and service delivery to the black and minority ethnic groups. One study found that the minority ethnic population underuse the hospices (Rees, 1986). Some explanations offered for this trend are that it could be a result of the tradition which exists within the Asian population of caring for the sick at home (Bhalla and Blakemore, 1981), or, as others claim, because the elderly wish to return to their country of origin to die when they have been diagnosed as terminal (Rees, 1990). A study commissioned by Cancerlink (Baxter, 1989) to examine palliative care services concluded that unmet needs of the black and minority ethnic patients and carers were due to communication difficulties, lack of information, inappropriate services and fear of discrimination.

Religious Composition of the City of Leicester

As discussed above, Leicester is a multiracial, multicultural city with one of the highest overall proportions of black and minority ethnic populations in the country. It has a variety of religious groups, each with different practices, principles and doctrines. A survey conducted in Leicester found that 66.1 per cent of the population were Christian, 13.9 per cent Hindu, 4.3 per cent Muslim, 3.8 per cent Sikh, 0.2 per cent Jewish and 12 per cent with no expressed religious belief (Survey of Leicester, 1983).

Methodology

A pilot study, using semi-structured tape-recorded interviews with six patients and carers, was initially undertaken by the first author to identify the key issues. This led to the development of a structured interview schedule which was then administered to a sample of 33 palliative care patients and carers from the BME groups.

Interviewees were recruited from various sources. All black and minority ethnic interviewees on existing client lists were selected from the voluntary sector and hospices. Those selected from the hospital were recruited over a two-week period by approaching all black and minority ethnic patients and carers attending radiotherapy and oncology outpatients clinics at one trust hospital in Leicester.

Unless otherwise stated, all results are based on 33 respondents.

Results

Cohort Description

All interviewees were resident in the City of Leicester at the time of interview. Nine patients and 15 carers were female. They had lived in the UK for 20 years or more. Twenty-one were Asian, Black Caribbean or Indian. Mean age for patients was 53 years and for carers 36 years. One patient and two carers refused to give their ages (tables 5.2 and 5.3). Most patients were at an advanced stage of their disease indicating that referral to some if not all of the services would have been appropriate.

Table 5.2 Length of residence in the UK

Years	patients n=15	carers n=18
10	2	0
11 – 20	2	5
21 – 30	9	7
31 – 40	2	5
Don't know	0	1

Table 5.3 Ethnicity of respondents

Ethnic Group	patients n=15	carers n=18
White	1	0
Black Caribbean	1	6
Indian	3	6
Pakistani	1	0
Chinese	0	1
Asian	9	5

Information and Communication

Gujarati was the main language for 20 patients and carers and English was spoken by 26 patients and carers. Those who spoke no English were interviewed in Urdu, Punjabi or Hindi by the first author.

Although 17 patients and carers interviewed felt they were able to find out most things about their illness as and when they wanted to, 18 patients and carers felt that there were things that they would have liked to be better explained.

Respondents were asked whether they required translation facilities – that is, an interpreter for speaking and/or reading written material. Although the majority of patients and carers said they did not require translation (25) or interpretation (29) facilities, one-third of patients and carers (10) said they preferred written material in a language other than English.

In response to questions about their GP, most respondents were positive towards their GPs. Most patients and carers claimed that their GP was willing to help (20), do home visits (19), sympathetic (20) and easy to contact (17). A number of patients and carers reported that their GP did not have enough time to talk (13) and that they did not have positive perceptions of their experiences. For example one carer, concerned about his mother, was met with the comment from his GP, 'What do you expect, she's got cancer' (resp 1). Another carer commented that, 'Because I used to ask, I felt as if I was a villain. I shouldn't be asking was the attitude' (resp 2).

Effective communication helps the patient and carer relax in otherwise difficult situations. One illustration of this was from a carer who attended outpatient clinics with his mother. The patient spoke no English, but became more relaxed and at ease when met by a nurse who spoke small phrases in Gujarati. Although the nurse could not have a conversation with the patient, her efforts and caring attitude clearly had a positive effect.

The level of adequacy of the information provided was addressed by asking patients and carers whether they had received information regarding their illness or services in a language which they felt was appropriate. Twenty-four patients and carers said they had not. Respondents who had received information did not generally feel that their questions had been answered or that the information was timely:

'The only way we received any information about the diagnosis was by writing to national organisations. We got no information about local organisations and found out about [the local hospice organisation] through our GP at the very last stage' (resp 6).

'I would have liked a better explanation of the diagnosis and some reassurance in plain simple English, if nothing else' (resp 8).

Occasionally, information provision was not the only problem. Coupled with that was the language and manner in which it was given. Patients reported that:

'With one foot out of the door, he [doctor] told me, "Oh, your cancer's spreadable"' (resp 9).

'I needed someone at the hospital to talk to when I was told I had cancer. I was sent a psychiatrist. I'm not mad' (resp 4).

'She [the patient] gets all wound up and concerned and she comes away and she clearly needs to have a detailed sort of information of what they said and put her mind at rest' (resp 10).

Service Access

Patients and carers were asked whether they were advised about particular services whilst a patient/carer, and whether they used any services during this time. Respondents reported that they had received little advice about the services that were available. At best, half of the respondents knew about hospital wards, outpatients and social workers. They were not advised about community services, the local hospice organisation and its services, daycare and voluntary services. Carers appear to have been more knowledgeable because they were more likely to speak English.

Table 5.4 Which of the services were used?

	patients (n = 15)			carers (n = 18)	
	yes	no	don't know	yes	no
Comm. Nurse	5	9	1	6	12
Macmillan Nurse	3	11	1	4	14
LOROS Nurse	1	13	1	2	16
M. Curie Nurse	0	14	1	0	18
LOROS	0	14	1	2	16
Hospital wards	6	8	1	7	11
Outpatients	7	7	1	6	12
Hospice care	1	13	1	0	18
Home care/help	2	12	1	3	15
Social worker	3	11	1	5	13
Day centre	1	13	1	3	15
Vol. services	3	11	1	2	16

These findings were further endorsed by the following extract from the interviews:

HHI: Did they tell you anything about the services that were on offer?

RS4: No, not really. But only the Macmillan nurse, she told, you know? Said everything, she told me all that. When I was told that I've got cancer, they said I've got to go to [the Leicestershire Hospice], and er, I might die there.

HHI: Who told you that?

RS4: Because they can't, they can't do anything about it.

HHI: Who told you about [the local hospice]?

RS4: It was this English doctor . . . I tell you, I was shocked like, like anything. I was crying all the time.

HHI: And is that all she told you about [the local hospice]?
RS4:   Yes.

Another patient said:

HHI: Did they mention any services at all that were available?
RS11:   No, none at all, none at all, no, nothing.
HHI: Were you offered any form of counselling or anything?
RS11:   No, no.
HHI: Would you have liked that?
RS11:   Well, I suppose so, I would. Nothing. I wasn't told anything. Nothing at all. As I said earlier on about other people, you learn, you know. When you speak to other people, you hear of other people getting help and you think, 'Why didn't that happen to me?' you know. Why didn't I get support like other people? It makes me bitter. I am bitter. I don't show it, though.

When asked how she found out about a voluntary support group, one carer replied:

'I had to drag the information out of the nurses. I kept asking them, "Look, where do I go from here?" after we were given the results, but they weren't forthcoming with the information.'

(resp 2)

However, once people do become aware of the services and enter the system, the service they receive is invaluable to patients and carers. As one carer commented:

'Information like that [about the hospice, Macmillan] was easy for me to get (a) because I was aware and (b) when I did ask people, they were very good at arranging things and arranging them quickly. We didn't have to wait for weeks or days because we were terribly concerned . . . and I wanted to get systems and help and support set up very quickly. I knew that my mother was going to be on her own and terribly frightened with not being able to communicate and be in control.'

(resp 10).

Religious and Dietary Requirements

Religious and dietary requirements are important parts of everyday life particularly so for the black and minority ethnic groups studied (Henley, 1982; Donovan, 1986; Helman, 1990). One indication of whether service providers have considered the needs of black and minority ethnic groups is to assess how well religious and dietary requirements are being catered for. Almost half of the patients and carers to whom such considerations applied (12/26) felt that an attempt was made to accommodate their dietary requirements while in hospital. However the majority of those who had stayed in hospital felt that no attempt was made to accommodate their religious requirements (18/27). One patient asked for a priest before her surgery, but was sent one after the event. She awoke to find herself being given the last rites by an Anglican vicar. The patient was a Roman Catholic. Another patient asked for an ordinary menu having been offered the 'ethnic' selection and she met with the comment from a nurse, 'Well, if you lot aren't going to bother eating them, what's the point in us lot providing them?' In the community, one elderly patient had, after much persuasion, agreed to receive the meals on wheels service. She had informed the services that as a Muslim she ate only Halal foods but wanted only vegetarian meals sent to her. The first meal that arrived was pork sausages. As a result, the patient refused to accept meals on wheels and the partially blind elderly husband was left to care and cook for his wife.

Racism

Patients and carers were asked, 'Did you experience any racism during your treatment in hospital?' and 'Do you feel you were treated any differently by the hospitals/services used, because of the way you look or dress or appear?' Eleven patients and carers said they had perceived certain experiences as 'racism' and 14 patients and carers stated that they had been treated differently. These questions stimulated further spontaneous comments. For example, one patient referring to her hospital stay said, 'I usually don't have a chip on my shoulder, but as a black patient, it was awful,' while another commented that she felt 'very conscious of being treated differently because of the way we looked.' Another patient said, 'I was made to feel like muck – they all hated me, I don't know why,' and followed on to give examples of many incidents which she felt happened because of her colour. Indeed she said, 'They wouldn't have said all those things if I had been white.' One carer commented that, 'Just because we wear saris and Punjabi suits doesn't make us idiots' (resp 5).

Discussion

This study was designed to investigate and describe the experiences of people from black and minority ethnic groups with regard to palliative care. The descriptive nature excluded a systematic comparison with the white population. However the findings of this study were compared to available research evaluations of palliative care conducted with predominantly white populations.

This study has demonstrated some deficiencies in access to and provision of palliative care services to the black and minority ethnic communities in Leicester. There was a low level of satisfaction amongst the black and minority ethnic groups with only 50 per cent being happy with the information that was being provided and with services in general, a lower level than that found in other studies (Cartwright and Seale, 1994). There were also divisions within the group with 50 per cent indicating that things were unsatisfactory and the other half indicating that they were happy with the information and communication which was taking place, and rating the services as good to excellent. However when the services are actually accessed and used, the picture is still poor. The low level of service use (table 5.4) appears to be unrelated to the severity or nature of the disease and to reflect the inadequate provision of advice about the services available.

Access to services and provision of information rely on effective communication taking place between the service users and the providers. Unsatisfactory communication contributed to distress for many of the patients and carers interviewed. Cultural and language differences between service providers and users posed a formidable barrier to effective communication in several instances. There appears to be considerable scope for improved communication and utilisation of interpreting facilities.

There is a need for information, both verbal and written, about the illness and the services which are available, in the language of the patient's choice. A suggestion for the type of information that patients and carers require has been summarised in figure 5.1. The areas which require increased emphasis for the black and minority ethnic groups concern the illness, the physical and non-physical side-effects and the services.

This study suggests that for people from the black and minority ethnic groups who do not have English as a first language information about services and diagnosis is not being made available in the language of their choice. It is further advisable that the provision of translated materials should be accompanied by suitable support systems through which further information can be obtained. A recurrent theme emerging from the interviews was the need for support services at the point of diagnosis, particularly in the hospital setting. Development of such a service is a priority and would benefit all users.

In order to access services, people need to be made aware of the existence of services. The experience of respondents interviewed is that information about most services available in the community is not being made available. This could be due to a language barrier which prevents effective verbal communication or to the provision of unsuitable leaflets, again because of inappropriate language. Another possibility, as with other populations, is that information is just not being made available.

In general, family and community networks appear to be stronger in the black and ethnic communities, and there is a tradition for caring for the sick at home amongst Asian groups (Bhalla and Blakemore, 1981). This has been used as an

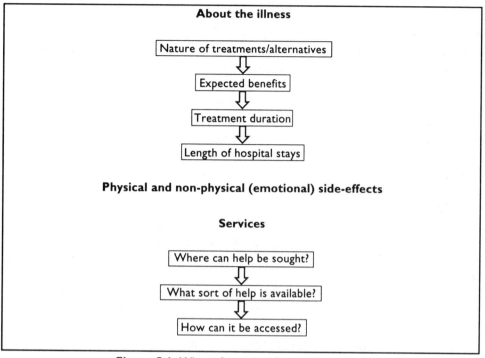

Figure 5.1 What information do people require?

explanation for underuse of support services. The extent to which this applies today is not known. Changing social and economic factors are determining where the younger generation live and more people from black and minority ethnic groups are moving away from the family. Hence the stereotype that 'they look after their own' is not always valid for this group of patients and carers and the reasoning has been called into question in a recent study (Baxter, 1989). The consequence is that people who require support and assistance are 'slipping through the net' (Webb Johnson, 1991).

The findings of this project suggest that current patient and carer support services in the community could be improved by becoming more accessible and culturally sensitive to the needs of the black and minority ethnic groups. The voluntary sector could have an important role in meeting some of these needs by offering social support and befriending services. However, the idea of support groups as portrayed by the voluntary sector is an alien concept to many members of the black and ethnic minorities. A support network could be established within existing black groups based in the black and minority ethnic community setting.

It has been claimed that institutional racism is one of the main reasons for unequal access to services by the black and minority ethnic communities (Burke, 1984; Fernando, 1984; NAHA, 1988; Ahmad, 1993; Alladin, 1992). Several of the patients and carers interviewed were extremely distressed because of racism. This highlights the importance of professionals being sensitive to and knowledgeable about racial and cultural issues. They need to be aware of how racism affects the lives of black and minority ethnic groups and alter their behaviour accordingly. Race-equality training for health care staff could prove to be a way forward. For example, information sessions and literature relating to death and bereavement issues, diet and culture would be invaluable to the care provider.

Many people were reluctant to say that they had experienced racism, almost to the point that doing so indicated some weakness within themselves. The reluctance among these groups to admit to being 'victims' of racism perhaps stems from the fear of recriminations for complaining. Racism is not a topic which is acknowledged or directly addressed, nor is the concept of racism a comfortable one. It dehumanises and disempowers. The reluctance is also due to the fact that it is rarely addressed. People are not used to questions about it. Perhaps those respondents who said they had not experienced racism had a lowered ability to recognise an experience as racism because they are living in a eurocentric society which is claimed to be equal.

The concern was raised in the report *Health for Leicestershire* (1993) which stated that:

'One key issue for the Black and Asian communities is the continuing presence of both overt and covert racism and discrimination within society. Racism like poverty is an important cause of inequality and injustice. Health and social care workers must be sensitive to racism and discrimination and take appropriate measures to remove them and prevent recurrence whenever and wherever they are identified.'

In conclusion it can be said that, in all the dimensions of care studied, communication, information, access to services and racism, there appears to be considerable scope for improvement. Although based on Leicestershire, the findings might have implications for any city in Britain with a significant black and minority ethnic population.

Acknowledgements

The authors wish to acknowledge the assistance of the following:

Leicestershire Health Authority,
Fosse Health Trust, Leicestershire,
Coping with Cancer, Leicester.

References

Adelstein A M and Marmot M G (1989) The health of migrants in England and Wales: Causes of death. In: Cruickshank J K and Beevers D G *Ethnic Factors in Health and Disease* pp.35–47. London: Wright.

Ahmad W (1993) *Race and Health in Contemporary Britain.* Buckingham: Open University Press.

Alibhai Y (1986) Culture shock. *New Society* **78**:11.

Alladin W J (1992) *The Politics of Race and Health.* Bradford: Race Relations Research Unit, University of Bradford.

Anthias F (1992) Connecting 'race' and ethnic phenomena. *Sociology* **26**:421–38.

Balarajan R and Raleigh V S (1992) Ethnic population of England and Wales 1991 Census. *Health Trends* **24**(4).

Baxter C (1989) *Cancer Support and Ethnic Minorities and Migrant Worker Communities*: Research Survey. London: Cancerlink.

Bhalla A and Blakemore K (1981) *Elders of the Ethnic Minority Groups.* Nottingham: Russell Press.

Burke A W (1984) Is racism a causatory factor in mental illness? *International Journal of Social Psychiatry* **30**(1 and 2):1–3.

Cartwright A and Seale C (1994) *The Year Before Death.* Aldershot: Avebury.

Cole M (1993) 'Black and Ethnic Minority' or 'Asian, Black and other Minority Ethnic': A further quote in nomenclature. *Sociology* **27**:671–3.

Cruickshank J K and Beevers D G (1989) *Ethnic Factors in Health and Disease.* London: Wright.

Dobson S (1983) Bringing culture into care. *Nursing Times* **79**(6):464–6.

Donaldson L J (1984) Occurrence of cancer in Asian and Non-Asian groups. *Journal of Epidemiology and Community Health* **38**:203–7.

Donovan J (1986) *We Don't Buy Sickness, It Just Comes.* London: Gower.

Fernando S (1984) Racism as a cause of depression. *International Journal of Social Psychiatry* **30**(1 and 2):41–9.

Fernando S (1988) *Race and Culture in Psychiatry.* London: Routledge.

Health for Leicestershire Annual Report of the Director of Public Health, 1993.

Helman C (1990) *Culture, Health and Illness,* 2nd edn. London: Wright.

Henley A (1982) *The Asian Patient in Hospital and at Home.* London: King Edward's Hospital Fund for London.

Higginson I (1993) Palliative care: A review of past changes and future trends. *Journal of Public Health Medicine* **15**:3–8.

Hopkins A and Bahl V (1983) *Access to Health Care for People from Black and Ethnic Minorities.* London: Royal College of Physicians.

National Association of Health Authorities (NAHA) (1988) *Action Not Words.* Strategy to improve health services for black and ethnic minority groups. Report of the National Association of Health Authorities. Birmingham: NAHA.

Office of Population Censuses and Surveys (OPCS) (1991) *County Monitors.* London: OPCS. (Series CEN 91 CM 1 – CEN 91 CM 54).

Parker H, Botha J L and Haslam C (1993) *Racism Experienced in the NHS.* Unpublished report, University of Leicester.

Rees D W (1986) Immigrants and the hospice. *Health Trends* **18**:89–91.

Rees D W (1990) Terminal Care and Bereavement. In: McAvoy B R and Donaldson L J (eds) *Health Care for Asians*. Oxford GP Services No 18, 304–19. Oxford: OUP.

Shaukat N, DeBono D P and Cruickshank J K (1993) Clinical features, risk factors, and referral delay in British patients of Indian and European origin with angina matched for age and extent of coronary atheroma. *British Medical Journal* **307**:717–18.

Survey of Leicester (1983) *Volume 1 – Initial Report of the Survey*. Leicester: Leicester City Council.

Webb P (1982) Health problems of London's Asians and Afro-Caribbeans. *Health Visitors* **54**:141–7.

Webb Johnson A (1991) *A Cry for Change: An Asian Perspective on Developing Quality Mental Health Care*. London: Confederation of Indian Organisations.

Westwood S, Couloute J, Desai S, Matthew P and Piper A (1989) *Sadness in my Heart: Racism and Mental Health*. Leicester: Leicester Black Mental Health Group and University of Leicester.

Chapter 6
Policy Issues and Provision of Cancer Services

Sue Hawkett

The views expressed in this chapter are those of the author only and not necessarily those of the Department of Health.

This chapter will consider the way in which health policy for cancer and palliative care has developed over the last few years and how this has influenced the provision of services. In tracing the development of cancer and palliative care services, the author will identify some of the major reports culminating with the current (August 1994) consultative document *A Policy Framework for Commissioning Cancer Services* (EAGC 1994). Although many of the reports have influenced Paediatric Oncology, this chapter does not deal specifically with children.

In order to put these documents and the development of policy into context, it is important to set them into the overall changes that have occurred in the NHS.

The last three years have seen major organisational restructuring to support the implementation of three White Papers *Caring for People*, *Working for Patients* and *Health of the Nation* (DoH, 1989a; 1989b; 1992).

As a result of the health service changes in 1991, District Health Authorities (DHAs) are charged with the responsibility of assessing the health needs of their population. They then contract with service providers to meet those needs in an effective and balanced manner, taking into account the views of the population they serve. The development of GP fundholding has enabled GPs to assess the needs of their patients and contract with service providers for care. Both DHAs and GP fundholders, however, have to take account of available resources when contracting services and to date GPs are able to contract only for certain services. The purchasers of health care have been encouraged to integrate primary and secondary care purchasing, to support the drive towards decentralisation in the NHS and develop stronger health authorities better able to champion the interests of local people (DoH NHS Management Executive, 1993b).

With the proposed merger of DHAs and Family Health Services Authorities (FHSAs) (subject to legislation) and closer working relationships with GP fundholders and local authorities, the potential for effective purchasing power will be enhanced. Such agencies will have the ability to take a strategic view of the resource requirements for cancer and palliative care (as for other services), thus identifying gaps and preventing over-provision and duplication. A possible danger of the merger of purchasing authorities is that of size, making it difficult to maintain effective communication between service providers and users. The Department of Health is working to reduce the danger. Clinical Nurse Specialists have a significant role to play in facilitating these links. In order to achieve this, nurses will need to transfer knowledge from an operational level to a strategic framework and provide advice to commissioning agencies (DoH NHS Executive, 1994).

Demand for Cancer Services

After coronary heart disease, cancers are the most common cause of death in England. There are over 200 different types of cancer and one in three people will develop cancer at some time in their life. Cancer is particularly predominant in older people. The cancer registration data for 1988 (England and Wales) showed that 65 per cent of new registrations were in people aged 65 or over (1.2 per cent under 25). Mortality data for 1992 showed that nearly 75 per cent of people who died from cancer were aged over 65, and 44 per cent were aged over 75.

In an average health authority with a population of 300 000, there would be about 1500 new cancer registrations and about 900 deaths from cancer each year (Association of Cancer Physicians, 1994).

The commonest cancers are shown in table 6.1.

Table 6.1 1988 Cancer statistics registrations, England and Wales, (OPCS)

Men		Women	
Lung	26%	Breast	26%
Non-melanoma skin	14%	Non-melanoma skin	13%
Colorectal	13%	Colorectal	13%
Prostate	12%	Lung	11%

The development of policy

There have been recurring themes in a number of reports which have contributed to and shaped the provision of care. As early as 1984, a subcommittee of the Standing Medical Advisory Committee reported on acute services for cancer

(SMAC, 1984). The terms of reference for the group, chaired by Professor Bagshawe, were:

> to consider the organisation of acute hospital services for the diagnosis and treatment of cancer and to make recommendations.

Size of the problem

Cancer is a major cause of death and avoidable ill-health accounting for about 25 per cent of deaths in 1992. It is predominantly a disease affecting elderly people. The increasing number of elderly people in the population has contributed to an increase in the demand for inpatient services, which has also been brought about by changes in treatment practices and development of preventative measures and early detection.

There is a growing public recognition that many of the common cancers, which may be difficult to treat in their later stages, are curable if detected and treated at an early stage.

Over the years, public awareness of the impact of early diagnosis and optimal treatment on the outcome of the disease has changed the level of expectation about what constitutes acceptable standards of care. There is an expectation and acknowledgement that the highest standards of treatment, including the latest developments, should be available to all.

The concept of equality of access is far from new and has been reiterated frequently. The 1970 Central Health Services Council annual report recommended that:

> an oncology service should be developed to ensure that all those in specific geographical areas had access to equal and high standards of care, generally but not necessarily within their broad locality, subject to the limitations of resources and general priorities.

The SMAC report (1984) argued that before services could be planned effectively, there was a need to consider the meaning of terms such as 'equal access to care', 'high standard of care', 'limitations of resources'. Ten years later, in 1994, the Association of Cancer Physicians, in a review of the pattern of cancer services in England and Wales, stated that the expectations of cancer patients were 'justifiably increasing', but claimed that the essentials of a cancer service were not provided uniformly. The report argued that with relatively straightforward planning a substantial improvement in quality and delivery could be achieved.

Access

In addressing access, it is necessary to consider the following:

- the cost of providing all types of cancer care within a reasonable distance of the patient's home;
- the extent to which professional staff in every hospital will have expertise in treating all kinds of cancer;
- the need for specific expertise when dealing with rarer forms of cancer;
- the wisdom of treatment for common cancers being concentrated in a small number of hospitals.

The Expert Advisory Group was set up to advise the Chief Medical Officers of England and Wales on the organisation of cancer services and to make proposals for advice to purchasers of cancer care. Its report describes one of the principles which should govern the provision of cancer services as that:

all patients should have access to a uniformly high quality of care in the community or hospital wherever they may live to ensure the maximum possible cure rates and best quality of life (EAGC, 1994).

The Association of Cancer Physicians (1994) stated that, from a national stand-point, access to modern resources and expertise was poorly coordinated and poorly integrated and the service lacked the structure to facilitate comprehensive evaluation or the implementation of new developments in a uniform fashion. The report proceeded to highlight the main problems facing the provision of cancer care and to suggest ways in which medical oncology could contribute towards their resolution.

Standards of care

The SMAC report (1984) stated that patients should be offered the most appropriate therapy in the light of current medical knowledge, taking into account the stage of the disease, age and general health. The report stressed the importance of a firm diagnosis being confirmed without delay. Delays are distressing for all concerned, and can be detrimental to long-term outcome. Also important was the requirement to give consideration to the needs of the patient in relation to the quality of life. Similar themes have been reiterated over the years in a number of documents from such bodies as the Department of Health (the Patient's Charter, 1991), Royal College of Nursing (1991), Joint Council for Clinical Oncology (1993), The Royal Marsden Hospitals NHS Trust (1994), Cancer Relief Macmillan Fund (1994), Royal College of Nursing (1993) and EAGC (1994).

The EAGC (1994) consultative document develops this theme, stating as a general principle of cancer care that patients, families and carers should be given clear information and assistance in a form they can understand about treatment options and outcomes available to them at all stages of treatment from diagnosis onwards.

Resource availability

The SMAC (1984) report stated that the NHS could not be insulated from economic realities. The resources allocated need adequately to reflect the very large number of patients affected and a sensible balance of provision between different aspects of specialised diagnostic and therapeutic services. It is recognised that the prevalence of cancer is likely to rise and will continue to do so for the foreseeable future. The Association of Cancer Physicians (1994) commented that the changing structure of the NHS, the increasing tendency towards specialisation and the awareness that resources are finite lend some urgency to developing a plan for the provision of cancer services across the nation.

Surgery

In 1984 it was stated that 30 per cent of the work of surgeons was the management of cancer (SMAC, 1984). The surgeon might be a generalist or one with a particular interest in management of certain types of cancer. The EAGC report (1994) has developed this theme in its recommendation that in a Cancer Unit (designated unit within a district general hospital undertaking the care of the commoner cancers), surgical management of cancer patients should be carried out by surgeons who specialise in a particular anatomical area.

The advantage of specialism is the accumulation of experience in complex procedures and high throughput of patients.

Radiotherapy

The SMAC (1984) report stated that it was preferable for patients undergoing radiotherapy to be cared for in designated radiotherapy beds staffed by nurses and medical staff experienced in their management. Again this theme has been reiterated and strengthened in such reports as SMAC (1991), Royal Marsden Hospitals NHS Trust (1994) and EAGC (1994).

Chemotherapy

It is generally acknowledged that chemotherapy has improved the survival rates for some cancer patients. The SMAC (1984) report noted that the relative ease with which chemotherapy could be used could lead to it being administered by doctors who, from the nature of their practice, did not have the extensive specific experience necessary for the optimum use of the drugs. The report claimed that there were marked differences between hospitals in the quality of results obtained with relatively routine chemotherapy.

This and other subsequent reports have maintained that to achieve optimum results doctors and nurses must have adequate training and experience and that it is essential for most chemotherapy to be administered under the supervision of doctors properly trained and specialising in its use. In 1989, the RCN Oncology Nursing Society produced guidelines for the safe practice with cytotoxic agents. They stated that:

Any nurse whose job involves cytotoxic agents, whether in preparation, reconstitution, administration, caring for the patient receiving therapy or dealing with disposal of body fluids or equipment, should have received training and assessment.

(RCN, 1989)

The Joint Council for Clinical Oncology produced a report on *Quality Control in Cancer Chemotherapy* in 1994. In it they state that:

It is clear that a method of treatment which is complex and which readily gives rise to life-threatening toxicity should be managed and administered by doctors and nurses with training and expertise in the field, in an unhurried environment where the procedures are carried out on a regular basis and with adequate checks on safety at every stage.

The Royal Marsden Trust, in their guidance on purchasing and providing cancer services, indicate target times for starting regimes for urgent, intensive or palliative chemotherapy (Royal Marsden Hospitals NHS Trust, 1994). The EAGC (1994) report recommends that chemotherapy should be given only in a specified location or locations in a hospital supported by specialist staff, particularly clinical nurse specialists in oncology nursing and other cancer nurses. The report goes on to argue that the provision of non-surgical cancer care scattered throughout hospitals and administered by a range of different disciplines is potentially dangerous and should be discouraged.

Role of the nurse

The nurse is in frequent and immediate contact with the patient and the focal point for the continuity of care. She/he makes a significant contribution in reducing the anxiety of the patient. Therefore it is imperative that she/he is well informed about the patient's treatments.

It is often the nurse who is asked for clarification by the patient. Considerable distress and loss of confidence can be caused if the nurse, whom the patient will see as a central figure in their care, seems to have little or no information on the treatment in progress.

The SMAC (1984) report recommends that, within a cancer unit, nursing care for inpatients at ward level and for outpatients should be planned and led by nurses who have benefited from post-registration education in oncology. The report goes on to state that the nursing service must be structured to ensure access to specialist nurses with site-specific experience. Nursing care in a cancer centre (designated centres for all cancers including common and less common cancers) should be planned and led by nurses with at least this level of qualification and experience.

Nurses working in primary care need not only the benefit of specific education and training, but also swift access to clinical nurse specialists who can provide advice and support.

Organisation of services

Services should always be developed to meet the needs of local populations. The problem with services being based on a relatively small number of comprehensive cancer centres is that they become isolated from the general health services at local district and community level and the burden of travel on patients and their families is increased.

The EAGC (1994) report has given advice on the organisation of cancer services and has made proposals for advice to purchasers of cancer care.

The new structure recommended by that group is based on a tier of expertise in cancer care as follows:

- **Primary care** is seen as the focus of care. Detailed discussions between primary care teams, units and centres would be necessary to clarify patterns of referral and follow-up to ensure the best outcomes.
- **Designated cancer units** should be created in many district general hospitals. These should be of a size to support clinical teams with sufficient expertise and facilities to manage the commoner cancers.
- **Designated cancer centres** should provide expertise in the management of all cancers, including common and less common cancers by referral from cancer units. They would provide specialist diagnostic and therapeutic techniques including radiotherapy.

Priorities and Planning Guidance for the NHS: 1995/96 (EL(94)55) states that as a success criterion for improving accessibility of care that:

Cancer services are purchased so as to provide the best possible quality of care for individual patients within the resources available. These should refer to the consultative report of the CMO's Expert Advisory Group on Cancer (EAGC, 1994) as appropriate.

Government initiatives

Prevention

The Government's long-term objective has been to reduce the mortality and morbidity caused by all cancers. Prevention is a key element in the fight against cancer. The UK actively supports the *Europe Against Cancer programme* which aims to reduce the number of deaths from cancer by 15 per cent by the year 2000, through prevention, public information and education, training and the coordination of research.

Health of the Nation

This is a key Government strategy for the reduction of cancers. Targets were set for four cancers.

* **Lung**
  reduce death rate for lung cancer by at least 30 per cent in men under 75 and 15 per cent in women under 75 by 2010;
  reduce prevalence of cigarette smoking in men and women aged 16 and over to no more than 20 per cent by the year 2000;
  in addition at least 33 per cent of women smokers to stop smoking at the start of their pregnancy by the year 2000;
  reduce consumption of cigarettes by at least 40 per cent by 2000;
  reduce smoking prevalence in 11–15-year-olds by at least 33 per cent by 1994.

* **Breast**
  reduce rate of breast cancer deaths in the population invited for screening by at least 25 per cent by 2000 (from 1990).

* **Cervix**
  reduce incidence of invasive cervical cancer by at least 20 per cent by 2000 (from 1990).

- **Skin**
  halt year-on-year increase in incidence of skin cancer by 2005.

Screening

National screening has been introduced for two cancers (breast and cervical). The case for screening for other cancers (e.g. ovarian, colorectal, prostate) has not been establis'._d. Screening should be introduced only where evidence suggests that early detection will make a difference to outcome, where an effective screening technique can be found and where effective treatment can be given once cancer is detected. The Department of Health is pursuing research in screening both through its own centrally commissioned programme and through the new NHS Research and Development programme. Health promotion and prevention of disease comprises one of the major themes of research, and one priority component of this theme is screening which includes a continuing commitment to the evaluation of cancer screening, in particular for breast and cervical cancer.

Health Technology

Health technology assessment has been given priority within the work of the NHS Research and Development Programme. The term 'health technology' is used to describe any method used by health professionals to promote health, prevent and treat disease, and improve rehabilitation and long-term care (DoH, 1994c).

Some of the present priorities for health technology assessment for cancer include screening for colorectal cancer, prostatic cancer and screening for melanoma.

Cancer Registration

The national cancer registration scheme in England and Wales is based on 11 Regional cancer registries in England and one in Wales. Cancer registries collect and process raw data (diagnoses, deaths etc.) and pass an agreed set of data to the Office of Population Censuses and Surveys (OPCS). OPCS validate these data and publish figures.

Health of the Nation – Four Major Cancers

The White Paper concentrated on the four major cancers for which the toll in terms of ill-health and death are high and where prevention measures and health education could reduce the mortality and morbidity significantly.

Lung Cancer

Primary lung cancer is the most common form of malignant disease in the western world. Because the disease is so lethal, incidence figures from cancer registration are closely related to mortality. In 1992, deaths from lung cancer amounted to 33 633 (22 639 male, 10 994 female). It is the most prevalent cancer among men over 65.

Screening
No useful screening method exists, so it is rarely possible to detect lung cancer before the onset of symptoms.

Prevention
Because of the close link between smoking and lung cancer, prevention can be achieved by educating the public on the effects of smoking, helping people to stop smoking, and protecting non-smokers from passive smoking. Those exposed to potential occupational hazards have a greatly increased risk if they also smoke. Awareness of occupational exposures associated with lung cancer, such as exposure to radioactive minerals, asbestos, nickel, chromium, coal gas, metallic iron and iron oxides is important.

The Chief Medical Officer's Annual Report for England in 1994 stated that progress had been made in three of the four main *Health of the Nation* targets related to adult smoking. Adult prevalence had fallen from nearly 30 per cent in 1990 to some 28 per cent in 1992. Over the three years to June 1993, total consumption of cigarettes had fallen by around 10 per cent compared to 1990. The proportion of women smokers who stop smoking at the start of their pregnancy was moving towards the target of one in three.

There was less success in teenage smoking. The levels amongst 11–15-year-olds were not reducing and had remained virtually unchanged. The Government were continuing their health education programmes targeted at young people, but the report pointed out that an important factor in success would be through family example.

Good Practice
The Standing Medical Advisory Committee Working Group on Lung Cancer has published guidance on current clinical practices in the management of lung cancer (SMAC, 1994).

By promoting key principles, the report aims to improve the standards of care and treatment of individuals with lung cancer throughout the country and to ensure that resources are used for maximum patient benefit in a cost-effective manner.

It is well known that the GP's role is crucial in the care of people with lung cancer. Early referral to a specialist is desirable to identify at an early stage those for whom curative treatment is appropriate.

The report stressed that the aim of the clinical management of lung cancer is to achieve a good quality of life for the person for as long as possible. Good symptom control and palliative care are now accepted as an integral part of the overall management of people with lung cancer, as with other life-threatening diseases.

A vital part of palliative care, which general practitioners and the primary care teams may share with specialists such as a chest physician or a palliative care physician, and voluntary organisations, is to act as a source of advice and support to the patient and the family as well as attending to the physical needs of the patient in terms of control of pain and other symptoms.

(SMAC, 1994)

Breast Cancer

Breast cancer is the leading cause of death from cancer in women over the age of 35 in Western Europe and North America. Each year in the UK some 25 000 women will contract the disease and 16 000 will die from it. In 1991 there were about 13 000 deaths in England, 89 per cent occurring in women of 50 years and over. Analysis of data from recent randomised studies demonstrates survival benefit among premenopausal women receiving chemotherapy and in postmenopausal women receiving adjuvant endocrine therapy.

Screening
In 1987 the Government launched a nationwide breast screening programme based on computerised call and recall at a cost of £70m. It is estimated that regular screening of women aged 50–64 should eventually save 1250 lives per year in England. This is the first programme of its kind within the EU and one of the first in the world. Good progress has been made in early detection which offers a better chance of effective treatment.

The key *Health of the Nation* target for breast cancer is for a reduction in the death rate for female breast cancer by at least 25 per cent in the population invited for screening, by the year 2000. The CMO's report predicted that by the end of 1993, 93 per cent of all eligible women would have received an invitation for screening. Although encouraging (71.3 per cent in 1992/93), take-up rates for screening vary from area to area, with as much as 80 per cent compliance in some suburban and rural areas to as little as 50 per cent in some inner city areas in 1993.

The NHS Breast Screening Programme published quality assurance guidelines in 1992 which aimed to ensure that patients were neither over-treated, with unnecessary mastectomies, nor under-treated, as judged by recurrence of cancer at the original site.

Before the NHS Breast Screening Programme began, very small cancers were rarely found. Surgeons have had to acquire new techniques for treating these early cancers. The guidelines built on what had been learnt over the first few years of screening to ensure that all surgeons working in breast screening could bring their practice up to the standard of the best.

(NHS Breast Screening Programme Review, 1994)

Good Practice

In 1994, Cancer Relief Macmillan Fund produced a leaflet on minimum standards of care for breast cancer. The standards include prompt referral by a GP, time targets for a confirmed diagnosis, information and choice regarding treatment and access to a specialist breast care nurse. Many of these issues are taken up in general terms in the EAGC (1994) report.

Cervical Cancer

Cancer of the cervix is a common gynaecological cancer occurring worldwide. It is the single most common cancer for women in the developing world. Although less serious in the UK it still accounts for the deaths of some 2000 women each year.

Screening

In 1988, the UK was the first country within the European Community to introduce a call/recall system for cervical cancer screening. This is designed to detect abnormal cells before they become cancerous and enable treatment to prevent cancer occurring. Most cervical screening is undertaken in GP surgeries and in 1990 a system of target payments was introduced for GPs who screen women aged 20–64 on their practice lists. Older women are recalled through the call/recall system if their previous two smears were not clear.

The eventual success of the screening programme will be measured by reduced cervical cancer incidence. The key *Health of the Nation* target is to reduce the incidence of invasive cervical cancer by at least 20 per cent by the year 2000.

Screening coverage increased in 1991/92 to 80 per cent of eligible women compared with 74 per cent in 1990/91. Maintenance of this high level of coverage means that the target reduction of 700 lives per year should be achieved. However, as with breast screening, high uptake in many areas may mask lower uptake in metropolitan areas. In 1993 the NHS Executive asked purchasers to set local programmes and targets for improvement (DoH, 1993a).

The quality of the programme is also important. The Chief Medical Officer and the Chief Nursing Officer wrote to all GPs and practice nurses reminding them of the need to ensure training and competency in such tasks as taking cervical smears (DoH, 1993b). Also EL(94)33 (DoH, 1994b) gives guidance on quality issues including refresher training for practice nurses.

Skin Cancer

Malignant melanoma is an uncommon but aggressive form of skin cancer. Once it has developed, half those affected will die from it.

Non-melanotic skin cancers, on the other hand, develop more slowly, occur mainly in old age, are relatively simple to treat and are rarely fatal.

The *Health of the Nation* target is to halt the year-on-year increase in the incidence of skin cancer by 2005. Three main objectives are identified for this to be achieved:

- to increase the number of people who are aware of their own skin cancer risks factors and, in the light of that knowledge;
- to persuade people at high risk to avoid excessive exposure to the sun and arti-ficial sources of ultraviolet radiation for themselves and for their children through the adoption of appropriate avoidance behaviour and sun protection measures;
- to secure an alteration in people's attitude to a tanned appearance.

(DoH, 1993a)

Palliative Care

Palliative care is an essential and integral part of effective cancer care. It can be provided in a variety of settings – in the community, hospital, hospice and nursing home. It is, however, from hospices that much of the knowledge, skill and motivation for change has emanated in supporting cancer patients and their families.

Palliative care is a multidisciplinary activity which crosses professional boundaries between health and social care. The needs of patients facing a life-threatening illness are multifaceted and may be shaped by a variety of personal, social and cultural factors. Palliative care principles can support people at different points of their illness and need not be confined to the terminal stages.

The National Council for Hospice and Specialist Palliative Care Services, which represents services in England, Wales and Northern Ireland, offers the following definition:

Palliative Care, as the World Health Organisation has recognised, is the active, total care of patients whose disease no longer responds to curative treatment, and for whom the goal must be the best quality of life for them and their families.

Palliative Care is now a distinct medical speciality in the United Kingdom. It focuses on controlling pain and other symptoms, easing suffering and enhancing the life that remains. It integrates the psychological and spiritual aspects of care, to enable patients to live out their lives with dignity, as well as offering support to families both during the patients' illness and their bereavement.

(Hospice Information Service, 1994)

In January 1994 there were 203 hospice/palliative care units operating in the UK and the Republic of Ireland with a total of 3110 beds, 573 of which were provided by 50 NHS units. There were approximately 370 home care teams, about two-thirds of which were attached to NHS hospitals. There were well over 200 day units.

A survey conducted by the Hospice Information Service and published in the 1994 directory, showed that in the UK almost 100 000 patients, principally suffering from cancer, were seen at home by palliative care nurses. This is well over half of all patients dying of cancer (160 000 die per year).

The EAGC report (1994) recognises the contribution and significance of palliative care as an integral component of cancer care. It stresses the importance of each district having access to specialist primary care and hospital/hospice-based services. The interdisciplinary palliative care team should contain trained specialist nursing and medical staff, to include social work, physiotherapy, occupational therapy and relate to other disciplines such as dietetics and chaplaincy (EAGC, 1994). Palliative care has developed through hospices, which has meant that it has grown in a rather ad hoc fashion depending on voluntary effort and fundraising. The EAGC report (1994) recognises this as a reason for links with health authorities being underdeveloped in some areas. The report recommends that where new developments are proposed, providers consulting with purchasers must have identified the local needs to ensure that services are not duplicated and most importantly that current services are being utilised.

Summary

This chapter has identified some of the significant reports from the profession or professionals advising the Department of Health, which have informed and shaped policy and influenced the provision of services. The Government has responded and showed its commitment to reducing the mortality and morbidity of cancer, particularly in relation to the four major cancers which cause the most ill health and death for which preventive measures can make a difference. The present EAGC (1994) consultative document will again inform policy and support subsequent changes in the provision of cancer services in England and Wales.

References

Association of Cancer Physicians (1994) *Review of the Pattern of Cancer Services in England and Wales*. Southampton: Southampton General Hospital.

Cancer Relief Macmillan Fund (1994) *Minimum Standards of Care for Breast Cancer*. London: CRMF.

Central Health Services Council (1970) *Annual Report for 1970*. London: HMSO.

DoH (1989a) *Caring for people*. Heywood, Lancs: Health Publications Unit.

DoH (1989b) *Working for Patients*. London: HMSO.

DoH (1991) *The Patient's Charter*. London: HMSO.

DoH (1992) *Health of the Nation: A Strategy for Health in England*. London: HMSO.

DoH (1993a) *Health of the Nation Key Area Handbook. Cancers*. London: Health Strategy Unit.

DoH (1993b) *Professional Responsibility, Accountability and Delegation of Tasks*, PL/CMO(93)14;PL(CNO)(93)6. London: DoH.

DoH (1994a) *Priorities and Planning Guidance for the NHS: 1995/96*, EL(94)55. London: DoH.

DoH (1994b) *Quality in the Cervical Screening Programme*, EL(94)33. London: DoH.

DoH (1994c) *Standing Group on Health Technology: 1994 Report*. London: DoH.

DoH NHS Executive (1994) *Building a Stronger Team: The Nursing Contribution to Purchasing*. Heywood, Lancs: Health Publications Unit.

DoH NHS Management Executive (1993a) *National Cervical Screening Programme* HSG(93)41. Heywood, Lancs: Health Publications Unit.

DoH NHS Management Executive (1993b) *Purchasing for Health: A Framework for Action*. Speech by Dr Brian Mawhinney. Heywood, Lancs: Health Publications Unit.

EAGC (1994) *A Policy Framework for Commissioning Cancer Services: Report by the Expert Advisory Group on Cancer to the Chief Medical Officers of England and Wales*. London: EAGC.

Hospice Information Service (1994) *1994 Directory of Hospice and Palliative Care Services*. St Christopher's Hospice, 51-59 Lawrie Park Road, London SE26 6DZ.

Joint Council for Clinical Oncology (1993) *Reducing Delays in Cancer Treatment*. London: Royal College of Physicians.

Joint Council for Clinical Oncology (1994) *Quality Control in Cancer Chemotherapy*. London: Royal College of Physicians.

NHS Breast Screening Programme Review (1994) National Coordinating Team, Fulwood House, Old Fulwood Road, Sheffield S10 3TH.

Office of Population Censuses and Surveys (OPCS) (1988) *Cancer Statistics Registrations: England and Wales*. London: OPCS.

Royal College of Nursing (1989) *Safe Practice with Cytotoxics*. London: RCN.

Royal College of Nursing (1991) *Standards of Care: Cancer Nursing*. London: RCN.

Royal College of Nursing (1993) *Standards of Care: Palliative Nursing*. London: RCN.

Royal Marsden Hospitals NHS Trust (1994) *Purchasing and Providing Cancer Services: a Guide to Good Practice*. London: Royal Marsden Hospitals NHS Trust.

SMAC (Standing Medical Advisory Committee) (1984) *Acute Services for Cancer: Report of a Working Group*. London: HMSO.

SMAC (Standing Subcommittee on Cancer of the Standing Medical Advisory Committee) (1991) *Quality Assurance in Radiotherapy*. Heywood, Lancs: Health Publications Unit.

SMAC (Standing Medical Advisory Committee) (1994) *Management of Lung Cancer*. Heywood, Lancs: Health Publications Unit.

Chapter 7
A Case Study of Early Detection of Cancer in the Older Adult
Catherine Evans and Alison Richardson

Introduction

In less than 40 years the percentage of older adults making up the British population is predicted to increase from 16 per cent to 18 per cent (Cancer Research Campaign, 1992). Since approximately 50 per cent of registered cancer cases and 60 per cent of all cancer deaths occur in this age group (OPCS, 1993a,b), this projected increase will inevitably lead to more cases of the disease (approximately 40 000 each year). In Britain, strategies attempting to reduce these statistics, in relation to lung, breast, skin and cervical cancer, are embodied within the White Paper *The Health of the Nation* (DoH, 1992). Regarding older adults, the Paper places emphasis on the role of primary health care teams to promote primary and secondary cancer prevention. This is a challenge to primary care, as a notorious feature of older adults who experience cancer is that they delay seeking medical advice until the disease is at a late stage (Yancik *et al*, 1988). Although this phenomenon is well documented, it is an area that has received minimal research. Little is therefore known about either the role primary health care plays in the failure to detect cancer at an early stage in this age group, or what motivates and inhibits older adults in reporting potential symptoms of cancer. This limited understanding would seem to be a major constraint on improving the nation's health.

The overall purpose of this study was therefore to explore both the role of the primary health care team and older adults' health behaviour in relation to early cancer detection. This dual perspective was intended to produce a greater understanding as to why older adults present with advanced cancer.

Background to the study

The value of early detection is undisputed because, after site of origin, the stage to which the cancer has advanced at diagnosis is the most important determinant of treatment (Holmes and Hearne, 1981). Early detection consists of two main strategies, namely:

- raising public awareness of early warning signs, so they can detect these themselves and access medical facilities for diagnosis and treatment;
- mass screening of the population to detect cancers in asymptomatic individuals.

(Corner, 1993)

Studies conducted in this area have predominantly considered the value and outcome of mass screening programmes. Such studies have revealed that only the mass screening procedures for breast and cervical cancer (i.e. mammograms and cervical smears) reduce mortality rates (Miller *et al*, 1991; Oddone *et al*, 1992). Although work in Sweden and Iceland has demonstrated that inclusion of women over 64 years in breast (Tabar *et al*, 1985) and cervical screening programmes (Johannesson *et al*, 1982) reduces mortality from these cancers, in Britain this age group is not routinely invited to attend screening.

Overall, the early detection of cancer in older adults relies upon both older adults recognising and reporting potential cancer symptoms, and health professionals enquiring about such symptoms during routine contacts.

In practice the few American studies which have looked at cancer detection in primary health care described the situation as one of 'missed opportunity' (Celentano, 1989) and in relation to nursing practice, older adults were the least likely to be offered cancer screening (Warren and Pohl, 1990). No studies have concerned themselves with British nursing practice in primary health care and cancer detection.

Causes of this delay or underscreening of older adults are suggested in the anecdotal literature to be possibly related to ageist attitudes held by health professionals and/or their attributing cancer symptoms to old age or chronic illness (Weinrich and Nussbaum, 1984; Dellefield, 1988; Given and Given, 1989). Again little research has concerned itself with the rationale behind health professionals' practice. All that is understood, consequently, is the presence of an age-related trend in offering screening, but little research-based explanation of why this occurs.

Early detection is quite obviously a two-way process between health professional and client. To promote early detection it is crucial to understand the reason why older people delay in reporting significant symptoms.

High health perceptions, education level and income were reported in a recent and seminal American study by Zabalegui (1994) to have a significant impact on older adults utilising available screening. Level of education was also found by Weinrich and Weinrich (1986) to be a predictor of cancer knowledge, along with race. In addition, the fear of cancer is frequently cited in the anecdotal literature as a major barrier (Weinrich and Nussbaum, 1984; Robbie, 1989; Given and Keilman 1990), but no research-based studies have directly examined older people's attitudes towards screening. This limits our understanding as to the extent and nature of this barrier, and moreover how nursing care can be directed to overcome it.

In general the early detection of cancer is an area of health care that has received minimal attention from either British or American nursing research. This means that although late-stage disease presentation in older adults is well documented, there is little understanding of why this phenomenon occurs. The aim of this study was therefore to begin to describe, in a systematic manner, strategies utilised in primary health care to detect cancer at an early stage in older adults, and to explore the promoters and inhibitors of this two-way process.

The study sought to answer three questions, namely:

- In primary health care what is offered to older adults to enable cancer to be detected at an early stage?
- What inhibits health professionals from including secondary cancer prevention activities in their practices when working with older adults?
- What influences and constrains the health practices of older adults in relation to early cancer detection?

Design and methods

In view of the limited literature in this area of health care it seemed prudent in a preliminary and descriptive study to reveal the opinions, attitudes and perspectives of both the lay public and professionals. To include the multidisciplinary team approach in primary health care a multi-focus study – covering general practitioners, health visitors, district nurses and practice nurses – was designed. To incorporate this multiple perspective the study was conducted in a health centre in North London.

Given the nature of this setting and subject matter the study was based upon a qualitative case study design. A case study design was selected because it enables the phenomenon to be investigated within its natural setting, using multiple sources of evidence (Yin, 1989). In addition a qualitative research approach lends itself to inductive reasoning, necessary in a preliminary study.

The multiple sources of evidence included eight of the 18 members of the health centre's primary health care team and 10 individuals aged between 65 and 85 years registered with the practice. Utilising convenience sampling to select the GPs and practice nurses, and purposive sampling for the health visitors and district nurses, two health professionals were drawn from each of the four disciplines working within the health centre. For the older respondents a simple random sample technique (Polit and Hungler, 1991) was used to obtain twenty names from a computer printout of the 1894 people aged over 65 years registered with the practice. Individuals with a history of cancer or who were mentally or cognitively impaired were excluded from the study. Fourteen informants agreed to participate, but because of constraints of time and resources only the first eleven were interviewed. Ten interviews were used in the final analysis.

The data collection instruments employed comprised two interview schedules (older respondents and health professionals), field notes to add to the depth of the description and supplementary questionnaires related to each group's biographical details.

Semi-structured interviews were used as the main method of data collection. For the health professionals, in an attempt to focus their responses within their professional framework, these were conducted in the health centre. In contrast, to maximise the older respondents' comfort, interviews took place in their own homes.

To make sure that the recording of this in-depth method of enquiry (Smith, 1975) was accurate, the interviews were audio-taped and then transcribed for analysis. A pilot study conducted with two informants, a district nurse and a 65-year-old man, made it possible to modify the researcher's interview technique and data collection instruments.

In order that the study could be related to previous theory, and in keeping with a case study design (Yin, 1989), interview probes were based upon topics developed during the literature review. Health professional interviews pertained mainly to the provision of and attitudes to secondary cancer prevention. The older respondents' interview schedule, with wording suited to 'lay' informants, maintained essentially the same topics.

Before data collection began, an informed consent was obtained from all respondents using an ongoing process (Munhall, 1988), which meant that they were given multiple opportunities for consent clarification and to withdraw from the study. To minimise emotional distress, the researcher adopted an open stance about the nature of the enquiry so that informants could withdraw at an early stage (Lee, 1993).

The researcher was also concerned that because of the health professionals' small sample size their anonymity would be difficult to maintain. This problem had been reported by Burgess (1985) using a single case study design in educational research. Health professionals were hence invited to censor the preliminary findings to ensure that they were accurately represented. Although this could be viewed as a limitation of an accurate rendering of the findings, Hammersley and Atkinson (1983) assert that such censorship enables respondents to confirm the perceived 'truth' of the experience, thus enhancing the study's validity.

The main limitation of this study design was that it consisted of a single case study of one particular health centre, chosen on the basis of its convenience to the researcher. This prevented comparisons being drawn between cases. The conclusions drawn from the study need to be viewed in the context of this limitation. In addition, no observations of the health centre were carried out as part of the study, so the data presented are retrospective and self-reported.

Results and discussion

The aim of this section is to provide a coherent and readable appraisal of the study's findings in relation to the research questions cited at the beginning of this chapter. To answer these questions, findings and analytical discussion are merged and in keeping with a case-study design are related to the research previously discussed (Yin, 1989). Further research is utilised to substantiate discussion where appropriate.

From the analysis of the 18 transcribed interview tapes, nine themes emerged (table 7.1) which fell naturally into the areas of the research questions. These are discussed under the headings, early detection – constraints in primary health care, influences on older adults' health behaviour and barriers to promoting cancer awareness in older adults.

Table 7.1   Prominent themes mentioned by respondents

Theme	Respondent
Psychological constraints on utilising information about cancer	Older Adult
Personal experience of cancer (friend or relation had had cancer)	Older Adult
Perception of health	Older Adult
Perception of cancer	Older Adult
Older adults' attitudes	Health Professional
Constraints on providing secondary cancer prevention	Health Professional
Cancer prevention	Health Professional
Knowledge about cancer and early warning signs	Older Respondent
Opportunistic and routine strategies to promote health	Health Professional

Early detection – constraints in primary health care

Table 7.2 provides a summary of what the primary health care team offered to their older clients for detecting cancer at an early stage. These findings are compared with Canadian and British guidelines. Issues surrounding the health professionals' adherence to British DoH guidelines (DoH, 1992; 1993a) will be discussed as this section unfolds.

Demographic details were obtained from the health professionals to establish potential influences on practice. Although professional experiences were diverse, no apparent differences were revealed in service provision or attitudes to practice.

The health professionals were invited to discuss how they incorporated health promotion, in particular secondary cancer prevention, when working with their older clients. Opportunistic strategies were identified as the most prominent approach ($n=8$). In addition four also mentioned using a routine approach, incorporated within a health check offered to the over-75s. Discussion about these approaches revealed a disparity of view among a small proportion of the nurses and the general practitioners as to the optimum way of promoting older adults' health.

The literature about health checks for the over-75s supports both viewpoints. Hastie (1990) suggests that health checks enable a comprehensive assessment to be made. In contrast, Tremellen and Jones (1989) and Hooper (1988) found that as primary health care teams already had regular contact with this age group, health checks were viewed as unnecessary and a more opportunistic approach of assessment during routine contacts was preferred. Indeed, Yancik *et al* (1988) advocate the value of opportunistic secondary cancer prevention because of older adults' regular contact with primary health care.

In this study, however, whether an opportunistic or routine approach was used, health promotion interventions were described predominantly in terms of 'giving advice' and centred mainly on the 'holy four' conception of health (McQueen, 1987) – diet ($n=4$), exercise ($n=3$), smoking ($n=3$) and alcohol ($n=1$). Given (1991) considers health promotion in relation to cancer as a health-orientated activity to detect early signs whilst maintaining well-being. In relation to cancer in men five of the health professionals stated their awareness of older men's risk of prostate cancer and incorporated discussion on continence issues when working with this age group. Offering older men information about prostate cancer was, however, mentioned by only a single health visitor.

In contrast to this awareness of prostate cancer, cervical and breast cancer prevention were described by five of the six nurses in terms of a 'forgotten' or 'neglected area' of their practice. This suggested that they were unaware of older women's increased risk of cancer, for as one district nurse commented:

'I've never thought about saying to someone when did you last have a smear and maybe you should have one . . . so that's a big blank in our practice.'

Lack of awareness as a constraint on providing cancer screening is supported by Warren and Pohl (1990) who, from the American perspective, found that this was a major reason why practice nurses did not offer older clients cancer screening. In this study, however, the majority of the nurses had cared for older women with breast cancer and subsequently seemed aware of the prevalence of the disease in

Table 7.2 Guidelines for cancer-related check-ups: A comparison between Canadian and British recommendations, and actual service provision

Condition	Canadian Recommendations*	British Guidelines	Health Centre's Service Provision
General cancer-related check-up	Annual health check providing information on primary prevention of cancer and examinations for cancers of the testes, thyroid, prostate, mouth, ovaries and lymph nodes.	Annual health check for those aged over 75 years, no specific guidelines on content (DoH, 1989).	Annual physical assessment – urinalysis, BP, weight, blood sample for anaemia, physical examination not routinely provided; social and psychological assessments for adults aged 75 years and over.
Breast cancer	Annual mammogram and CBE† after age 50 (A). Every 1–2 years between ages 40 and 49 (C). Monthly self-breast examination age <40 (C). Annual mammogram and CBE after age 60 (B).	Tri-annual mammogram for women aged between 50 and 64 years; breast awareness for women 65 years and over; mammogram on request for women 65 years and over (DoH, 1992; DHSS, 1986).	CBE† offered in 75-year health check and opportunistically by GP. Teaching breast awareness not routinely offered to women over 65; Mammogram offered to women over 65 when symptoms of breast cancer present (n=8).
Cervical cancer	Annual PAP tests from 18 years (B). After three consecutive normal smears, frequency performed at the discretion of the physician.	Five-yearly PAP tests for women from 18 until 64 years old. No further screening if three consecutive normal tests, and the last one performed no more than three years previously.	Cervical screening history not routinely checked; discussion and provision of PAP test not routinely offered to women aged 65 years and over.
Colorectal cancer	Less than 40 with no known risk factors – no routine recommendations. (C). Over 40 with no known risk factors – no routine recommendations, however evidence does not warrant stopping faecal occult blood testing (C).	No recommendations. Primary prevention – reduction in high fat foods and increase in starchy and fibre-rich foods (HEA, 1993).	No screening offered. Dietary advice (n=4).
Lung cancer	No recommendations.	No recommendations Primary prevention – smoking cessation (DoH, 1992).	Chest x-ray offered by one GP to adults with a smoking history – 'a gut reaction' not policy; advice on smoking cessation (n=3).
Prostate cancer	Annual digital examination for men (C).	No recommendations or primary prevention.	Digital rectal examination offered by one GP during 75-year health check; considering incorporating PSA‡ screening; opportunistic and routine urinalysis and assessment of continence change (n=5).
Skin cancer	Annual skin examination for men and women over 40 (D).	No recommendations. Primary prevention – avoid excessive sun exposure (DoH, 1992).	Issue not directly discussed, 2 nurses mentioned observing for signs on face and neck.

†CBE – Clinical Breast Examination; ‡PSA – Prostate Specific Antigen; * **Codes:** A There is good evidence to support the recommendation; B There is fair evidence to support the recommendation; C There is poor evidence that the recommendation is of value.; D No evidence to support recommendation. (Canadian Task Force Guidelines cited Baird et al 1991)

this age group. This suggested that they experienced (and cited) a number of constraints on cancer prevention in practice (table 7.3), and that explanations for under-screening were more complex than simply lack of awareness of the high incidence of cancer in older adults.

Table 7.3   Constraints on early detection

	Perceived constraints on promoting secondary cancer prevention	No. of Respondents identifying the theme
1	Lack of time (workload)	6
2	Patients' problems overwhelming	5
3	Providing information about cancer might arouse fear	3
4	Presence of physical barriers (re: PAP tests and BSE)	5
5	Screening not justified by research	3
6	'. . . something quite often forgotten about.'	5
7	Inadequate training on early cancer detection	5
8	Lack of facilities (re: teaching BSE)	2
9	Lack of client motivation	3
10	Information confusing (re: BSE or 'breast awareness')	4

A consistent theme that emerged as to why cancer prevention was not incorporated in the nurses' practice was the need for updating and further training. An EEC (1989) directive also highlighted this problem in its recommendations for inclusion of a greater emphasis on cancer prevention and detection in basic and post-basic nursing training.

Considering that among the older respondents six identified the health centre as a possible source of information about secondary cancer prevention, this training constraint on practice needs to be addressed. Moreover, at the national level the *Health of the Nation* guidelines lay emphasis on raising individual awareness to prevent cancer and detect at an early stage (DoH, 1992; 1993a). In the light of this study's findings this would seem unlikely without the creation of further training opportunities in this field of health care.

In addition to lack of training, the issue of older adults consulting for chronic health needs was raised by four of the nurses to explain the apparent 'gap' in their practice in offering older women cervical and breast cancer screening. Both practice nurses explained:

'I think it's a combination of their not coming in for a specific well women orientation, whereas if I have a cervical smear booked in I immediately go into a well women mode.'

'I tend not to [teach BSE] . . . because it normally goes along with the smear and because we don't smear ladies over the age of 65 we don't tend to teach self-breast examination.'

Chronic health needs acting as a barrier to practitioners offering secondary cancer prevention was suggested by Warren and Pohl (1990) and Celentano (1989) as an explanation for their finding of underscreening of older people. The findings of this study would appear to support their supposition.

As well as the practitioners citing individual constraints, organisational constraints of the health centre's protocols for cervical screening and the over-75s health check were highlighted. In relation to cervical screening, the health centre's position can be best explained by drawing upon the comments of one of the practice nurses who stated that:

'It wouldn't be a problem to recommend it [PAP test] . . . but obviously I have to work within the practice protocol . . . so I can't start saying to women over 65 I thought you ought to have a smear without the protocol changing . . . I probably wouldn't smear a patient over 65 only because that's how the protocol is really.'

This comment is of some concern, considering that DoH guidelines clearly state that:

there should be no upper limit for women who have never had a smear . . .

(cited Draper, 1982)

In fact, this study found that not one of the four female respondents had an adequate screening history. In addition, two of these women actually expressed that they would like to discuss cervical screening with a health professional.

Similarly, the finding that the practice nurses did not offer older women teaching on breast self-examination questions their familiarity and understanding of DoH (DoH, 1993a) guidelines which set out to advocate 'breast awareness' for women over 65. Some of the health professionals however appeared to be held back by confusion surrounding whether breast awareness or BSE should be incorporated in their practice and if either procedure was of any value. This apparent lack of clarity and research underpinning practice guidelines evidently needs to be addressed.

In relation to the health centre's protocol for the over-75s' health check both a practice nurse and a general practitioner described it in terms of being 'quite limited' and lacking in 'specific questions to raise people's awareness of cancer'. This seemed a 'missed opportunity' when both health professionals and older respondents identified that a function of the health check was the early detection of unrecognised problems.

The approach consequently adopted by the nurses to detect cancer appeared to be reactive, with only a general practitioner adopting a more proactive approach:

> *Health Visitor – reactive approach* 'I have to say it's not something we actually ask [breast lumps] . . . but the few that I've had have actually indicated that they had lumps.'
>
> *General Practitioner – proactive approach* 'I check their [men's] prostates for evidence of prostatic cancer . . . with my elderly women patients I always check their breasts for lumps.'

A proactive approach in secondary cancer prevention and older adults is important, considering that American studies have found that this age group have a very limited understanding of potential cancer symptoms (Weinrich and Weinrich, 1986), and a major reason for underutilisation of screening like mammography is lack of physician referral (Rimmer, 1993).

Although the general practitioner's comment appeared to suggest an active involvement in the health check, his comment was punctuated by:

> 'I see fewer and fewer people personally with regard to elderly screening . . . I'm not sure if that's good thing or not . . . I'm not sure if that [breast and prostate check] is always done . . . by the nurses.'

Discussion with the nurses involved in the health check revealed that physical examination was not performed by them. This apparent role-confusion was also evident in a general practitioner's and health visitor's comments in relation to not teaching BSE, who both stated that they referred older women to the practice nurse. This suggests that they were unaware that the practice nurses did not incorporate this in their practice when working with older women.

Such role-confusion is not uncommon in primary health care teams, even when, as in this case, the community nurses were attached and shared the same premises as the general practitioners (Bruce, 1981). For as Bowling (1987) states from her review of studies of primary health care teams, the most crucial question which the team ought to discuss openly is 'who does what'.

From these findings it seemed that role-confusion constrained the secondary cancer prevention services offered and should be addressed, particularly as examples of a cohesive approach in practice, described in a recent DoH paper (DoH, 1993b), have been seen to be a pivotal factor in the provision of primary health care.

Influences on older adults' health beliefs

The older respondents were aged between 65 and 85 years (mean 73.1 years) and comprised four women and six men. Socioeconomic circumstances and educational level varied from individual to individual (table 7.4). All but one of the respondents were retired. The majority (*n*=7) had known a close friend or relative who at one time had had cancer.

Table 7.4   Characteristics of the older respondents

Characteristic	No. of Respondents
Age Range	
65 to 85 years (mean = 73.1 years)	10
Sex	
Male	6
Female	4
Social Circumstances	
Live Alone	4
Council/Housing Association Tenant	7
Home Owner	3
Education	
9 years	5
10 to 13 years	5
Further Education	3
Professional Training	4
Ethnic Origin	
White (Irish)	1
White (Russian)	1
Mixed White/Afro-Caribbean	1
White (English)	7

Respondents were asked about their contact with the primary health care team at the health centre under study. The most frequent contact was with the general practitioners, with most respondents (*n*=9) consulting them during the last year and visiting the health centre on a regular basis (4–6 monthly).

Such terms as 'charming'. 'very helpful' and 'pretty good' were used by nearly all the respondents to describe general practitioner consultations. Probing of these comments revealed that activities of 'he listens' (*n*=5) and 'asks how I feel' (*n*=4) were viewed to be particularly useful. One respondent commented in relation to why this approach was helpful:

'They're more matey with you, they don't sit above you, like . . . they come down to your level . . . It makes it easier to communicate. I hate authority . . . I

don't like people dictating to you . . . The other way I wouldn't tell them a thing
. . . so they'd get nothing out of me.'

Considering the older respondents' regular contact with the health centre and take-
up of preventive health care when offered, this suggested that the general
practitioners' mode of communication facilitated service utilisation. Indeed Svarstad
(1986) showed how a non-authoritarian and a caring approach enhanced general
practitioner consultations, while an authoritarian approach resulted in older adults
concealing information.

Seven of the respondents, however, also identified that to consult a doctor in
general or if a potential cancer sign was experienced, symptoms needed to be either
considered as legitimate or to be persistent before they initiated consultation. This
point was reflected in the comments of two respondents:

'I don't really like going down there bothering him unless I think it is really
necessary . . . If it's aches and pains I wouldn't go down there . . . other things I
might.'
'Supposing I had detected blood . . . one might want to ignore it . . . if it
continued then you would go to the doctor.'

This suggests that delay in seeking medical advice may be associated with the
nature of symptoms experienced. Care, however, is required in the analysis of these
comments because they reflect anticipated behaviour rather than actual behaviour.
Yet one respondent actually enquired during the interview about possible presence
of skin cancer. As her comments illustrate, delay in symptom-reporting seemed to
be related to the nature of the symptom and previous consultations:

'I do have a bit over there [on face] which doesn't heal but I've never gone to the
[health centre] . . . it has been there for several years . . . I think it just indicates
my attitude to [the health centre] . . . I feel like I'm not seriously ill . . . I feel like
I have to be seriously ill before I go there.'

Two studies, one American (Rakowski et al, 1988) and the other British
(Williams, 1983), reported that active response to symptoms was more common if
they were persistent and in the case of Williams' study, symptoms were then
categorised into those that did and did not warrant medical consultation. This
provides some understanding as to why older adults may decide to delay symptom
reporting.

The older adults' attitudes towards preventive health care also varied within the
group. For two of the men take-up of advice on smoking cessation was viewed as
unnecessary for men of their age – 77 and 70 years. As one of them stated:

'I think it's a bit late for me now to start worrying about these things [smoking cessation], if I'd been 27 instead of 77 I might have took more notice.'

In contrast, three respondents, two of whom were aged 67 and the third 77, expressed that it would be useful to them if the health centre offered more preventive health care. Interestingly the three respondents who expressed the desire for more preventive health care to be offered had the highest educational level in the sample. In view of the similarity between the older respondents' age, the reason for the different attitudes to health and preventive health care may have been connected to the respondents' educational level. This is supported by Zabalegui (1994), who found that older adults with a high educational level had higher health perceptions and utilisation of preventive health care, compared to those with a lower educational level.

Variation between male and female respondents' attitudes towards secondary cancer prevention measures was less clear. For the women breast self-examination was performed by all four and was regarded as a simple procedure performed on 'a now and again' basis. The majority of the women had not received information on breast self-examination. Their awareness seemed to be derived from breast examinations performed by their general practitioner, as well as, in one case, from the media.

In contrast to the women's positive response about breast self-examination, views about mammography screening were mixed. These varied from lack of interest to anger, as reflected in the comments of two respondents:

'It's not something I'm interested in . . . if I knew a bit more about cancer it might interest me.'
'I'm involved with several older women's groups and they feel very strongly that . . . our health service is very wrong . . . because the incidence, ah . . . does not decrease over the age of 64 and they feel women over the age of 64 should be pulled in for treatment.'

Most of the health professionals (n=7) also had the view that the ceiling of 64 years should be raised. Two, however, reflected the first older woman's response of uninterest by stating:

'There's a lot of elderly people who will refuse it.'
'The trouble is getting them to go.'

This reflects the Government's main argument (DHSS, 1986) that mammography screening is not offered on grounds of low compliance. In this study three out of the four women thought a mammogram would be of value.

Attitudes towards cervical smears were a little more consistent. Of the three women who had never received a cervical smear cause for the absence of screening was equated to experiences as younger women. For two women this was because of 'gynae' surgery, and smears consequently were described in terms of 'I've never gave it a thought' and 'I'm unclear about it'. In neither case did the surgery performed contraindicate a cervical smear. The third woman commented:

> 'I haven't had one . . . They weren't regularly done when I was younger. It was never suggested but if it was I would.'

Cervical screening in the older women was apparently not done because they had not received it when younger. This gives support to the anecdotal literature in which a consensus is reached that older women have not been smeared because they were moving out of their child-bearing years at or around the time when the test was introduced, and so have not had contact with family-planning or obstetric care where the test is mainly offered and publicised (Dellefield, 1988; Blesch and Prohaska, 1991). To have smears now, as older women, would be a new experience, requiring recommendation by a health professional.

Male attitudes towards uptake of secondary cancer prevention were difficult to explore as no screening is specifically available. However, one respondent said that he would like to be offered a screening for prostate cancer, and a second for colorectal cancer. In both cases this was related to comments of 'It's in my own best interest to know.'

Promoting cancer awareness in older adults

Older respondents' knowledge of the causes of cancer was relatively accurate. Only one respondent mentioned the myth of cancer being caused by a knock or fall. Smoking and hereditary tendency were the most commonly cited; smoking was mentioned by all respondents and hereditary tendency by seven.

The predominant identification of smoking as a cause of cancer is in agreement with a larger British survey of adults' attitudes to and knowledge of cancer by the Cancer Relief Macmillan Fund (CRMF, 1988). The finding of the majority of older adults not expressing the myth of cancer being caused by a blow or knock, however, contrasts with an earlier American study (Weinrich and Weinrich, 1986), and the findings of the CRMF survey.

Eight respondents identified that information about the cause of cancer had been derived from the media, six of whom specifically cited the Health Education Authority's anti-smoking campaign. This suggests that current government efforts to reduce smoking (DoH, 1992; 1993a) had had some influence on the older respondents' awareness of cancer. This recent health education drive may explain why the cause of cancer was accurately identified to be smoking, as opposed to being identified as a myth.

Older adults' knowledge of cancer was also discussed in relation to their understanding of early warning signals. As was found in a larger American study

(Weinrich and Weinrich, 1986), knowledge of early warning signs was limited. The respondents, on average, could name only one or two of the Cancer Research Campaign's seven warning signals (mean=1.9) (table 7.5). Two respondents named four signs and one respondent was unable to name any. Again, the respondents who named the highest number of warning signs had the highest educational level, which supports Weinrich and Weinrich's (1986) findings. However, this was not a consistent finding, with one respondent of equally high educational level able to name only one sign. This suggests that the basis of utilisation of information about cancer is more complex than educational level.

Lumps were the most widely known early sign and were mentioned by eight of the ten respondents, again in agreement with Weinrich and Weinrich's (1986) study and the CRMF survey (1988).

The majority of respondents (n=6) mentioned the myth that pain was an early warning sign of cancer. A prominent influence of this misconception was that eight of the ten when asked about early warning signs described personal experiences of friends or family who had had cancer. This tended to mean that knowledge about cancer was described in terms of its late stage.

'I've had various friends who've had cancer. This young friend who has cancer, she's lost a lot of weight and she's in great pain she's having secondaries . . . ah, so any kind of persistent pain, I guess.'

No respondent had seen information on early warning signs. Four of the respondents identified that they did not want information unless they experienced cancer. Gentle probing of this attitude revealed that this was associated with a fear of cancer itself. This again tended to be rooted within the older adults' personal experience of cancer.

'I don't want to know about it unless it's necessary . . . I've seen people die from it. The less I know about it the better I feel because seriously if you know too much, you think, oh my god, I've got a bump here, I've got a pain there, maybe it's going to be cancerous.'

The fear of cancer was a prominent theme of the interviews and concomitant with this were negative perceptions of the disease and its treatment, with four respondents describing cancer using terms of 'It's a one way street', 'Once you've got it it's too late', and one saying:

'It's a terrible disease, cancer, people die of cancer every day of the week . . . People suffer, it's painful . . . they go through all kinds of therapy. I'd rather say good-bye than go through all that, I wouldn't want to mess about like that.'

Table 7.5 Older respondents' knowledge of early warning signs

	A change in bowel or bladder habits	A persistent sore throat, nagging cough or hoarseness	Unusual bleeding or discharge	Thickening or lump in the breast, testis or elsewhere	Persistent indigestion	Difficulty in swallowing	Obvious change in size or bleeding of mole	Pain	Weight loss
Respondents	2 Respondents	2 Respondents	2 Respondents	8 Respondents			4 Respondents	6 Respondents	3 Respondents
Quotes	'...blood in his motions...' '...how his bowels... and bladder work...' 'Blood in the urine'	'...a sore throat' '...a terrible cough...'	'...coughing up blood...' 'In the lungs... you bring up blood'	'Find a lump' '...a breast lump...' '...a lump first...' '...got a lump...' 'A lump somewhere.' '...women should examine their breasts...' '...lumpy breasts...' '...a lump in their breast...' '...a lump in her thyroid.'	NOT MENTIONED	NOT MENTIONED	'...a bit... which doesn't heal...' '...you get a bump.' '...a blemish at first...' '...sores or blotches on the skin'	'Pain presumably.' '...a pain here...' '...some sort of pain' '...some kind of pain' '...persistent pain...' '...you get pains from it...'	'...she's lost a lot of weight...' '...losing a lot of weight...' '...anorexia and possible weight loss.'

←——— Imperial Cancer Research Fund: Seven Warning Signals For Early Diagnosis ———→ ←— Early Sympton Cancer Myths —→

The image created during the interviews was that cancer was not simply a fatal disease but a metaphor for suffering, viewed as synonymous with death itself, and a death that involved much pain. This supports Sontag's (1979) argument that society has a distorted image of cancer. The finding, however, that cancer was synonymous with death is in contrast to the CRMF (1988) survey which found that although cancer was feared by a considerable proportion of the sample, 92 per cent agreed that some cancers could be cured. This contrast suggests that older adults' cancer attitudes may be more negative than the population as a whole and be based on the reality that the highest incidence of people who die from cancer occurs in this age group (OPCS, 1993a).

Considering the respondents' image of cancer, how misinformed they were about the disease, and that they chose, as one respondent expressed, to 'turn a blind eye' to such issues, this image is an evident and deep-rooted barrier to raising older adults' awareness of early cancer symptoms. Brooks (1979) supports this analysis, suggesting from an earlier survey of adults' cancer attitudes that the depth of fear revealed was so great it seemed to prevent individuals from seeking help for symptoms of cancer.

This present study's finding concerning older adults' fear and negative attitudes towards cancer – not aided by current health education strategies of emphasising 'risk' – supports Corner's (1993) view that a more positive message needs to be conveyed which emphasises that the quality of living with cancer can be improved with early diagnosis and treatment, and that this is the case even when the disease is incurable.

Conclusions

The aim of this study was to begin to throw light on why older adults are frequently not diagnosed with cancer until a late stage. The literature review revealed a number of areas that required investigating. These included the nature of secondary cancer services offered to older adults in primary health care and the constraints on health professionals in providing this. The review also pointed to the investigation of older adults' attitudes, perception and knowledge about cancer and what influenced their health behaviour.

This study was designed to answer these questions. The findings have revealed that, in the primary care setting under study, the provision of secondary cancer prevention was limited and contrasted with DoH guidelines. This gap in practice was found to be predominantly related to the precedence given to meeting chronic health needs, limiting time available to offer secondary cancer prevention. Even if these time constraints were addressed, a further barrier is nurses' lack of training in this area of health care. Within the multidisciplinary team, problems of collaboration and role confusion also constrained the provision of secondary cancer prevention.

With the older adults, their education level plus their health professional's communication style appeared to influence health beliefs and uptake of preventive health care. This complex interaction between health beliefs and health practices was one aspect which seemed to inhibit the take-up of secondary cancer prevention for this age group. In addition, the reality of the fear of cancer (rooted predominantly in its being viewed and experienced as synonymous with death itself) seemed a major barrier to the older adults seeking and utilising information about cancer. The prevalence of this fear and the extent to which it acted as a barrier would seem to raise the question whether mass screening of this age group holds the answer to reducing cancer mortality. Rather, a sensitive individual approach from a health professional offering opportunistic cancer screening would seem to be of greater value.

Before such practice recommendations can even be considered, further evidence is required to support this study's findings. To achieve this, the researcher suggests that the study be replicated on a far larger scale, incorporating multiple cases, to enable comparisons to be drawn across a range of primary health care settings. In broadening the study, it is advocated that to obtain a more representative perspective of primary health care the various models of care delivery are included. In addition, to explore educational and ethnic differences in older adults' knowledge of cancer, the researcher suggests approaching health centres in contrasting social settings, for example rural and inner-city centres.

In addition to provision, further research which might produce evidence to support this study is needed into older adults' fatalistic view of cancer. In particular, a comparative study between older adults and other adult age groups would be a useful contribution to this area of research. On the problem of insufficient training, the researcher suggests that a future initiative should involve researching and developing ways of tailoring the skills of primary health care teams to the needs of older adults. A sensitive individual approach of opportunistic screening during routine contacts would seem, in the light of this study, to be a possible way forward.

References

Baird S, McCorkle R and Grant M (eds) (1991) *Cancer Nursing: A Comprehensive Text Book.* London: WB Saunders.

Blesch S and Prohaska T R (1991) Cervical cancer screening in older women. *Cancer Nursing* 14(3):141-7.

Bowling A (1987) Teamwork in primary health care. *Nursing Times* **79**(48):56–9.

Brooks A (1979) Public and professional attitudes towards cancer: a review from Great Britain. *Cancer Nursing* 2(6):453–60.

Bruce N (1981) *Team work for Preventive Care.* London: John Wiley.

Burgess R (1985) *Issues in Educational Research: Qualitative Methods.* Lewes: Falmer.

Canadian Task Force in the Periodic Health Examination (1989) The periodic health examination update: 2, 1989 update. *Canadian Medical Association Journal* **141**:209–216

Cancer Relief Macmillan Fund (1988) *Public Attitudes to and Knowledge About Cancer in the United Kingdom*. London: Thornton Drummond and Brett.

Cancer Research Campaign (1992) *Cancer in the European Community Factsheets*. London: CRC.

Celentano D D (1989) Early Detection of Cervical Cancer. In: Yancik R and Yates J W (eds) *Cancer in the Elderly: Approaches to Early Detection and Treatment*. New York: Springer Publishing.

Corner J (1993) Health Promotion and Cancer Care. In: Dines A and Cribb A (eds) *Health Promotion Concepts and Practice*. Oxford: Blackwell Scientific Publications.

Dellefield M E (1988) Informational needs and approaches for cancer detection in the elderly. *Seminars in Oncology Nursing* **4**(3):156–68.

DHSS (1986) *Breast Cancer Screening: Report to the Health Ministers of England, Scotland, Northern Ireland and Wales* (working group chaired by Sir Patrick Forrest). London: HMSO.

DoH (1989) *Terms of Practice for Doctors in General Practice*. London: HMSO.

DoH (1992) *The Health of the Nation*. London: HMSO.

DoH (1993a) *The Health of the Nation: Key Area Handbook – Cancers*. London: HMSO.

DoH (1993b) *The Health of the Nation: Targeting Practice: the Contribution of Nurses, Midwives and Health Visitors*. London: HMSO.

Draper G J (1982) Screening for cervical cancer: revised policy. The recommendations of the DHSS Committee on Gynaecological Cytology. *Health Trends* **14**:37–40.

EEC (1989) Commission recommendation concerning the training of health professionals in the matter of cancer. *Official Journal of the European Communities* **32**:1–7.

Given B (1991) Compliance and Health Promotion Behaviours. In: Baird S, McCorkle R and Grant M (eds) *Cancer Nursing: A Comprehensive Text Book*. London: W B Saunders.

Given B and Given C W (1989) Cancer nursing for the elderly. *Cancer Nursing* **12**(2):71–7.

Given B A and Keilman L (1990) Cancer in the elderly population: research issues. *Oncology Nursing Forum* **17**(1):121–3.

Hammersley M and Atkinson P (1983) *Ethnography: Principles in Practice*. London: Tavistock.

Hastie I (1990) Assessment of the over 75s. *Horizons* **5**(4):258–62.

Health Education Authority (1993) *Cancer: How to Reduce Your Risks*. London: HEA.

Holmes F F and Hearne E (1981) Cancer stage-to-age relationship implications for cancer screening in the elderly. *Journal of the American Geriatrics Society* **29**:55–7.

Hooper J (1988) Case finding in the elderly: does the primary health care team already do enough? *British Medical Journal* **297**:1450–1.

Johannesson G, Geirsson G, Day N and Tulinius H (1982) Screening for cancer of the uterine cervix in Iceland 1965–78. *Acta Obstet Gynaecol Scand* **61**:199–203.

Lee R (1993) *Doing Research on Sensitive Topics*. London: Sage.

McQueen D V (1987) *Research in Health Behaviour, Health Promotion and Public Health.* Research Unit in Health Behaviour and Change Working Paper. Edinburgh: Research Unit in Health and Behavioural Change.

Miller A B, Chamberlin J, Day N E, Hakama M and Provok P C (1991) *Cancer Screening – UICC Project on Evaluation of Screening for Cancer.* Cambridge: Cambridge University Press.

Munhall P (1988) Ethical consideration in qualitative research. *Western Journal of Nursing Research* 10(2):150–62.

Oddone E Z, Feussner J R and Cohen H J (1992) Can screening older patients for cancer save lives? *Health Promotion and Disease Prevention* 8(1):51–67.

OPCS (1993a) *1992 Mortality Statistics: Cause of Death in England and Wales.* London: HMSO.

OPCS (1993b) *1987 Cancer Statistics: Registrations in England and Wales.* London: HMSO.

Polit D F and Hungler B P (1991) *Nursing Research: Principles and Methods,* 4th edn. Philadelphia: J B Lippincott.

Rakowski W, Julius M, Hickey T, Verbrugge L M and Halter J B (1988) Daily symptoms and behavioural responses: results of a health diary with older adults. *Medical Care* 26(3):278–97.

Rimmer B (1993) Improving the use of cancer screening for older women. *Cancer* 72(3):1084–7.

Robbie P W (1989) Cancer screening in the elderly. *Journal of the American Geriatric Society* 37:888–93.

Smith H W (1975) *Strategies of Social Research: Methodological Imagination.* London: Prentice-Hall.

Sontag S (1979) *Illness as a Metaphor.* London: Allen Lane.

Svarstad B L (1986) Patient–Practitioner Relationships and Compliance with Prescribed Medical Regimes. In: Aiken L and Mechanic D (eds) *Applications of Social Science to Clinical Medicine and Health Policy.* New Brunswick: Rutgers University Press.

Tabar L, Gad A, Holmberg L H, Ljungquist U, Fagerberg C J G, Baldetorp L, Grontoft O, Lundstrom B, Manson J C, Eklund G and Day N E (1985) Reduction in mortality from breast cancer after mass screening with mammography. *Lancet* (8433):829–32.

Tremellen J and Jones D A (1989) Attitudes and practice of the primary health care team towards assessing the very elderly. *Journal of the Royal College of General Practitioners* 39:142–4.

Warren B and Pohl J M (1990) Cancer screening practices of nurse practitioners. *Cancer Nursing* 13(3): 143–51.

Weinrich S P and Nussbaum J (1984) Cancer in the elderly: Early detection. *Cancer Nursing* 7(6):475–82.

Weinrich S P and Weinrich M C (1986) Cancer knowledge among elderly individuals. *Cancer Nursing* 9(6):301–7.

Williams R (1983) Concepts of health: An analysis of lay logic. *Sociology* 17(2):185–205.

Yancik R, Kessler L and Yates J W (1988) The elderly population: Opportunities for cancer prevention and detection. *Cancer* 62:1823–8.

Yin R K (1989) *Case Study Research: Design and Methods*, 2nd edn. Newbury Park, California: Sage.
Zabalegui A (1994) Barriers to health. *Nursing Times* **90**(1):59–61.

Section Three

Cancer and Personal Relationships

Chapter 8
The Experiences of Families of Newly Diagnosed Cancer Patients – Selected Findings
Hilary Plant

Introduction

This chapter will explore the ways in which people live with a diagnosis of cancer in a partner or parent or friend. It is based on one area of analysis from a research study of the experiences of family and friends of newly diagnosed cancer patients. The study revealed differences between the family and patient, not only in their experience of the illness but also in their perceptions and reactions to it, thus creating an additional burden on both and showing that both patient and family have to live with two levels of adjustment – dealing with their own reactions to cancer and also with that of others. However, it is the patient who is invariably offered a larger share of support from other family members or friends or from health professionals. As one woman who participated in this study, herself a patient, commented:

> 'All of the focus is on the victim, the focus is not on the family, and they've got to get through it. They are the ones who need the real help.'

Background to Study

Current philosophies of care include the family as well as the patient (RCN, 1991). However, as the patient's well-being is the priority for the professional carers, there is often little time to work out the intricacies of the family network. Assumptions may be made about how the relatives feel or should react, and when they do not conform they may be classed as difficult or simply ignored. The life of the husband of the woman quoted above had been radically changed by her illness. Yet, because of poor communication on the part of health professionals early in her illness, he did not visit the hospital, so unlike her he gained no support from the hospital staff.

A wide range of research studies and papers has been drawn upon during the process of this research, including literature on chronic illness, lay caring, social support and family studies. There are also an increasing number of studies specifically about the effects of cancer on other members of the family. However there is little agreement about what methods should be used to address this complex area. In the nursing literature Oberst, for example, has found that after surgery for cancer the spouse may be more distressed and certainly less well supported than the patient (Oberst and James, 1985). More recently it has been shown that the caregiving burden for patients perceived by professional carers as requiring little care may in fact be substantial for the family (Carey *et al*, 1991). Indeed it has been found that for some family members there is a significant decline in mental health status over time (Ell *et al*, 1988).

Several authors have addressed how cancer affects the whole family system and the role adaptation required in the family when one member becomes ill (Cassileth and Hamilton, 1979). Northouse, in a review published in 1984, divided the illness up into phases, with specific problems for the family just as there are for the patient (Northouse, 1984). This argument has recently been expanded (Sales, 1992). Both authors comment on the deficiencies they perceive in the research which has taken place to date. These are congruent with my own reading which indicates that, with the exception of the studies mentioned above, most data is collected on one occasion only, thus excluding the major part of the illness trajectory. Usually only one family member, most often the spouse, is consulted and research has concentrated on the partners of women with breast cancer and the parents of children with cancer. The studies are often not designed to allow an airing of issues that the family themselves may see as a problem.

Research Approach

The aim of this study was for participants to tell the researcher their own story about their life since someone close to them was diagnosed with cancer. The research has been designed to explore the experiences in context and to look at the complexity of the experiences and how they change with time. The approach taken to structure the data collection and analysis was based on grounded theory (Glaser and Strauss, 1967). Thus interpretation and analysis could begin from what was emerging from the data rather than from any preconceived idea, theory or hypothesis.

This study about family and friends was part of a larger project looking at cancer patients' perceptions of need (Bliss and Johnson, 1993). Thus for this study both patients and relatives were interviewed. Patients with cancer of the colorectum and lung were contacted three months after being told of their diagnosis and a home visit was made to find out if they would like to participate in the research. If consent was obtained a tape-recorded interview took place. At the end of the interview they were asked who they believed had been most affected by their illness and permission was sought to approach this person to take part in the study.

If those nominated by the patient consented to take part, they were interviewed at approximately three, seven and 13 months from the time when the patient was diagnosed. On some occasions, more than one person per patient was interviewed. Where possible, a bereavement interview was recorded at about three months after death if the patient died during the study.

Twenty patients and 26 relatives have been recruited into the study. No friends have been nominated; indeed, in this sample the family network appeared to be the most important social link. The relatives were a predominantly female sample, reflecting the fact that lung and colorectal cancers occur more often in men and that where the patients were married they all nominated their spouses first. All single patients nominated a woman, sisters not brothers and daughters before sons. This coincides with other literature about lay caring and families (Hicks, 1988).

The first interview with the family member was open, but focused around their thoughts and experiences from the time when they first thought that something might be wrong with their relative. Subsequent interviews gave an opportunity to develop rapport with the participants and more importantly to go back and test the ideas that had arisen and explore what they had meant in their previous interviews (Laslett and Rapoport, 1975). After some initial interviews I realised that much as I wanted the participants to be able to tell an unbiased account of what life was really like, my interactions with them could not help but influence the story they told and my interpretation of it. Thus a reflexive approach to the fieldwork was taken where there was a 'deliberate linking of social process of engagement in the field with the technical processes of data collection and the decisions that linking involves' (Ball, 1990).

After the interview a questionnaire was completed, covering details about the participant's own health and about their main sources of lay and professional support. They were also asked their reactions to taking part in the study.

I also recorded a commentary on my own thoughts and feelings about what went on in the interview. These data included reflections on my interaction and relationships with the participants, for example the issues that were difficult to talk about and what happened when the tape-recorder was turned off – in essence my perception of the subtext of the interview – which provided crucial contextual information for the analysis (Daly, 1992).

Process of the Research

To discuss the findings, first I will consider the process of doing the research and how this in itself illuminates the experience of the family.

The interviews recorded for this research have had a very profound effect upon me. The stories were often long and compelling and I became very involved with what the participants were telling me. The interviews revealed an enormous diversity in experience, in the way the experience was perceived and then in the way it was retold to me. The accounts ranged from extremely emotionally charged, through to flat matter-of-fact, from highly articulate to a series of 'you know what I mean's.

This study was conducted entirely in the homes of the participants. This setting was crucial because it was the experience at home which I was studying. I also believed that meeting people on their home territory would make them feel more at ease than if they were interviewed in hospital. Nonetheless, I was still the middle-class educated woman. I was not living with someone with cancer and I was thus necessarily in a more powerful position than those I was studying, who may have been careful about how they presented themselves to me (see Cornwell, 1984).

In the initial interviews I felt uncomfortable about intruding upon someone's already difficult life, asking them to recount their experiences for my tape-recorder, then thanking them and leaving. Feminist researchers (e.g. Oakley, 1981; Webb, 1984) are concerned about the power balance in the research relationship and believe that the research should benefit not only the researcher, but also the researched. In this study I decided that as far as I was able and in the knowledge that I had no access to medical records I would answer questions and give advice where I felt that I had the understanding to do this – the resulting interactions all becoming a crucial part of my data.

Nevertheless, having made this decision I was still constantly confronted by dilemmas. The participants in this research did not present me with straightforward questions about side-effects of treatment. On occasion I felt my face being searched for agreement as I was being told that they believed that their relative was going to be cured. Twice I was asked outright how long I thought that their relative had got to live. Although this was not difficult to deal with, as obviously I did not know, it was harder to hear accounts of poor care or mismanagement by the professionals.

It was paramount during the process of this research that the individual's resources marshalled for living with a diagnosis of cancer in a close family member should not be disturbed. There is a growing debate, particularly within nursing (Smith, 1992; De Raeve, 1992) about the implications of undertaking research to study human experience in distressing situations, especially where the research is of a qualitative nature 'sometimes evoking strong emotional responses and sometimes pursuing thoughts that might otherwise never be revealed' (Cowles, 1988). It is difficult fully to inform participants of the potential risks and benefits of taking part in the research, when at the outset the flexible nature of the research means one is unable to predict in advance exactly what the participant is going to say and therefore what effect this process is going to have upon them.

Potential benefits and risks of the research

The participants were often very enthusiastic about the research and many showed this with increasing hospitality as the study went on.

The majority of the participants said that they found the interviews helpful and valued the opportunity to talk about their experiences – often things they had been unable to mention to anyone else: for example their fears about the future and thoughts about what would happen to them if the patient died. One woman at her first interview started to cry and explained: 'It's actually the first time I've talked to anyone.' After her third interview, I asked her to comment on the effect that the interviews had on her. She said:

'I cried the last two times and I think it does you good. Afterwards you feel better that you've let the emotion out because somewhere that's been bottled up . . . I think you need to do it.'

There could be several reasons why participants felt they benefited from taking part in the research: the cathartic nature of the interviews which allow free expression of the situation; the therapeutic power of being listened to; the opportunity to voice fears without feeling judged and the 'helper therapy principle' where participants may allow themselves to talk about their problems because they perceive it as helping somebody else (Reissman, 1976).

There are drawbacks with this sort of research relationship, however. There is no therapeutic contract with the participant. So, whilst talking might temporarily offer some relief, something may be started which could then remain unfinished. Offering an outlet and then withdrawing could potentially be quite harmful as could the opportunity to reflect on something that the relative would rather not think about (La Rossa *et al*, 1981; De Raeve, 1992).

In this study I attempted to avoid problems by a careful negotiation of access at the first and all subsequent interviews, respecting the participant's level of adjustment as far as possible. A lengthy debriefing was undertaken at the end of each interview and the participant was also asked about the effect the interview had had upon them. A contact telephone number was always left, but this was only ever used by participants for updating me with news.

A second issue concerning consent was the initial explanation of the purpose of the research. After some early problems when gaining consent from patients recruited to take part in the main project, the diagnosis was not mentioned by the researcher until after the participant had made reasonably clear their understanding of the illness. This avoided disruption to those who may be coping with the illness by 'denial', or if where the relative was interviewed the patient had not actually told them that they had cancer.

Analysis of the Interviews

Grounded theory requires the fracturing of data to reveal common themes which may then be restructured into an analytical framework. I have identified a list of recurring themes from the initial interviews some of which are discussed below. However, I found it difficult to tamper with the stories which people told, as I was concerned about taking their words out of context (see Garrow, 1992; Darbyshire, 1994). I have therefore attempted in this chapter to reflect the nature of the whole story as well as focusing on particular issues.

The interviews which were conducted with the patients provide some of the context of the relatives' experiences. There seems to be a difference in style between the transcripts of the patient interviews and those of the family. The patients tend to provide a more direct description of events; they are telling their own story. Many of the relatives gave less focused interviews. They were in fact telling multiple stories. Even those most distressed about the illness and who talked about it in terms of 'we' and 'our' did not give such a clear linear account as the patients. These people found it hard to think about themselves. Some of them could not really see the point of doing research about their own experience at all, as it was the well-being of the patient which was paramount. On the other hand those perhaps less close to the patient were sometimes even harder to focus. For example, one daughter talked for nearly 45 minutes about her own post-natal depression and another woman talked for even longer about her father-in-law's suicide. The very stories that the relative participants told reinforce the idea that they are attempting to cope on more than one level.

At first I was rather disappointed by this. I wanted a clear picture of their difficulties which could then be addressed. However, on reflection, the way the relatives told their stories was providing the crucial contextual information that I had been so keen to keep in the research. The subordination of their own story and needs to those of the patient for some, or the burden of additional problems in their life for others, were indicators of the emotional pressure that the families were under and begin to illustrate why it is sometimes so difficult for health professionals to provide support.

Living with Someone with Cancer – Some findings

The data that have been analysed so far reveal a series of diverse and complex experiences. In this study the experience appears to be mediated by the participant's relationship with the patient, how the cancer is perceived by the relative and what else is happening in their own life at the time (cf. Given et al, 1988; Rolland, 1989).

The family invariably have to live not only with their own feelings about the illness and the expectations that they have of themselves in this situation, but also with the patient's way of reacting to the cancer, which may be at variance with their own. These interviews illustrate the relatives' ways of coping with the patients' way of coping (by coping I mean here the processes whereby 'the individual learns *how* to tolerate or *put up* with the effects of illness' (Bury, 1991). One of the features of both the patient and relative interviews is the way they reconstruct the future as a way of guarding against uncertainty. There often seems to be a need to plan out how events will unfold, perhaps to make them less frightening. It seems that patients and families also plot out what they think will (and sometimes should) happen. Del Vecchio Good *et al* (1994) describes 'therapeutic emplotment' whereby American physicians attempt to plot out the course of the disease for their patients in order to reduce the uncertainty. Patients and families also tend to do this, but sometimes they are not each constructing the same story.

Reconstructing the future

A common thread running through the interviews is the knowledge that a diagnosis of cancer, graphically described by one participant as 'the crack of doom', is a life-threatening event. Therefore both the patient and their family are forced at whatever level and however briefly to consider the prospect of the patient's death. One of the things that the relatives have to cope with on top of their own feelings about this is the patient's way of reacting to the news:

'He actually never thought he would, from the start, never ever thought he'd get through . . . from the first day he found he had cancer, that was it, and we had to go and make wills out.'

Families had to cope with a range of reactions. Some patients refused to mention the likelihood of death and the incumbent practicalities, such as making a will. Other patients, particularly those with lung cancer, made dramatic preparations for their death such as digging up and altering much-loved gardens, cutting down hedges that had taken years to shape and clearing out the precious contents of garden sheds – one man sold his boat, which his wife found particularly hard to bear because to her it represented her husband at his happiest. These relatives had to stand by and be supportive while the patient destroyed many years' work, sometimes the thing that was most dear to them and sometimes the things that the relatives wanted as a memory if the patient did die. In many instances it was the patient who determined how these practical things were going to be played and the relative had not only to cope with this but also to be seen to be coping. As one woman commented:

'I try to hold it in. And he's . . . I suppose what I try to do a lot is make him feel that I can manage.'

On occasion some relative-participants even seemed to use the interview process to show the patient that they could 'manage' the situation. The tone might change if the patient came into the room or sat in for parts of the interview. They used speaking to me to tell the patient that they could cope.

There was obviously a range of differences in approach to the situation seen in the study. Some couples professed to be 'coping together' while in others the illness created an almost unbearable tension. There was also a variation of degree in openness of discussion and similar coping styles did not necessarily mean ease in communication.

Residual separateness

Even in the couples who professed to have open communication, the relative often felt that they had to somehow carry the burden of their own grief and protect the patient from it.

One woman who was able to talk with her husband about death and was proud of how they shared things together still felt that she must hide her own sadness:

'But . . . no . . . I suppose now and again I have a cry . . . but I mean I'm on me own then. I don't . . . I suppose I don't hide things from him, but I wouldn't let him see me upset 'cos it would upset him. And you can't . . . well not . . . as he is, you can't . . . (G is very tearful again) . . . upset him. Oh I don't know. It does seem unfair, doesn't it?'
Interviewer: 'Yes'
I said to him, why can't we go together . . . that's the ideal solution, isn't it . . . because I'd be lost without him.'

Another man who almost physically wanted to bear his wife's illness for her tried to hide his own tears from her. He describes their relationship:

'I'm afraid we both feel almost together I mean I've been saying sometimes "we".'
Interviewer: 'Yes, I noticed.'
We empathise very much, um, and I have on occasion I suppose felt her symptoms. Um, I have for well a matter of some months now I have on more occasions than not had a feeling of stomach pain, now I'm quite clear in my mind that there's actually nothing wrong with my stomach.'

And soon after:

'I think almost every time, after she had gone out and I was on my own doing something I would quite often break down and cry, um, but she didn't realise that.'

Even in these couples which shared the experience quite closely there was a 'residual separateness'. These relatives seemed to feel that as they did not have cancer they could not always burden their loved one by showing them the acuteness of their own grief. Many of these are strategies for protecting the patient from any possible additional hurts. I called these strategies 'buffering' in an earlier paper (Plant, 1992).

Non-disclosers

Other couples appeared to have a joint strategy of dealing with the illness together by not talking about the cancer. As one man explained:

'We decided . . . the wife and I . . . well we won't, tell anybody . . . we'll just hope that's the end of it.'

They did not even tell their 36-year-old daughter who lived with them. This interview was for me one of the most difficult and distressing. The relative-participant, the patient's husband, described their relationship as close, and he had cared for his wife meticulously after her discharge from hospital. He told me:

'Having gone through that [surgery], you're just pleased it's over with, that's all there is to it.'

This participant was unable verbally to express any distress about his wife's illness to me. Yet throughout the interview there were tears streaming from his eyes. He did not allow me to acknowledge this or to stop the interview. It was as if he was having to play an 'everything is fine' role and could not allow any opportunity to ventilate his own emotions. I felt the research process itself was threatening to disturb his fragile balance and that it made sense when the couple very nicely told me that they did not want to undertake a third interview.

Others could not even allow things to go this far. One woman had to look after her father who came round to her house every day but had never been able to tell her that he had cancer. The first relative I asked to take part in the study refused. Her husband seemed surprised that I should even be interested in her well-being. When I told her about the research she started crying. She explained to me that she had been keeping it all inside her for so long and that she must keep going. It seemed it would be almost unbearable to focus on her own emotion. It was not that she was not interested in the research, indeed we developed such a good rapport when I was interviewing her husband that she phoned me the day after he died.

For these participants, however close they were to the patient, there was no opportunity even to begin to ventilate their emotions. They were devoted to the well-being of the patient and to them this meant not expressing how they felt. The relative did not want to show themselves to be more distressed by the illness than they jointly 'agreed' that there was reason to be.

The patient's way

Invariably the forms of coping were dictated by the patient even when they were said to be mutual. For example, one couple who lived within sight of their hospital were never allowed by the patient to leave the area, not even to visit their son in case something happened. Another woman was not allowed to visit her husband in hospital, although she went to stay with her sister who lived only a few streets away while he was in having treatment. Sometimes the relatives had to scheme to get what they wanted, such as accompanying the patient to outpatient appointments.

Unacknowledged burden

In the less 'close' relationships the relative often had to bear an even more unacknowledged burden. These were sometimes the siblings or children who were perhaps less involved with the day-to-day life of the patient but nonetheless saw themselves as responsible for caring for them.

As one participant, the sister of the patient, explained in tears:

'You feel you've done everything that you can and then you're just shut off from it when you feel you want to be there. And you want to say something, [but] you're not being given the opportunity to sort of say the right words. . .

'I think that's one of the hardest things is that when you feel you could be there for somebody they put up a barrier against you . . .

'You do feel guilty and I suppose really if you're very honest with yourself after a while (and this is the hardest thing in the world to say) you resent illness. And this sounds awful but . . . when someone's ill for a long time like that you do somewhere deep inside you begin to think, you know, um, you're never going to get better or, um . . . It's hard to explain, I suppose it's almost an intolerance after a while which you then feel terribly guilty about.'

Her employers threatened her with the sack if she took any more time off work to look after him. Yet when I talked to her brother about where he got his support from he said from the oncology unit and within himself. He said his family were over-sensitive and that they could not understand what it was like to have cancer. His sister had never been allowed to speak to any health professional about her situation except to me and the interviews she described as her 'therapy sessions'.

In the above quotation she is also illustrating one of the issues that came up in several of the interviews, that is the guilt and resentment that some of the relatives begin to feel about this intrusion into their life by the cancer and in the end sometimes also by the person with cancer. One husband of a woman with colon cancer explained that his life was 'on hold' and he felt unable to apply for a new job. This was, however, usually inadmissible within the relationship.

Supervision of activities

There seemed to be both active and more passive strategies taken by the relative to live with the patient's way of dealing with the illness. These put a varying degree of pressure on the relative to maintain them. Many were living with the same knowledge and distress as the patient, but felt that at least in their public reconstruction of the future they needed to maintain hope. One woman explains how she feels she actively has to make her husband cope.

'But I think the actual illness makes me tough, because I'm determined to get Arthur through it, although he is quite strong he's a very emotional person . . . and possibly not as strong as me and one of you has got to make the other one cope with it I think.'

In their striving to get things the way they think they should be, the relatives variously describe their roles as the 'bully', the 'villain' or the 'bogeyman'.

It was particularly the women in the interviews who seemed to be attempting to supervise the activities of their husbands. It involved attempting to prevent the patient from dwelling on what had happened to them by encouraging them to think about or do other things. For example several women felt that the patient should take up a hobby, join an evening class or take exercise. Sitting and thinking or watching too much television were considered bad.

For example one woman commented:

'Quite honestly, apart from being ill, he doesn't help himself, he'll sit and think about it.'

And later:

'But I just wished he would find an interest so it gets him out more.'

The women seemed to be aiming to protect the patient from themselves and organise them so that they would be more positive and not become 'down' and thus more vulnerable to the cancer. These are examples of the relative attempting to plot a course of the illness for the patient. However, they are having to use persuasion rather than more overtly planning how they think things should be.

Monitoring

This appeared in the interviews when the patient attempted to assert their independence and would not allow any more direct help from the relative. This led to a surveillance of the patient's environment to prevent any unexpected upset or intrusion by the cancer. One woman explained how she had become 'super conscious' about cancer and the media. She explained:

> 'I tend to scan the *Evening Standard* and look for all the things that might be on [about cancer] and try to watch the other side.'

It might also involve a constant monitoring of the patient's physical health, for example keeping a close watch on what they ate. The patient's general well-being might be assessed by looking at their facial expression and behaviour rather than by actually talking to them.

Nonetheless the relative's attempts at monitoring the patient could sometimes feel uncomfortable. One woman with colon cancer complained of feeling 'suffocated' by the way her sister manoeuvred around her need for independence despite her illness and increasing weakness. Another patient did not like his wife's muted discussions at the door:

> 'What's going on? I'm still the superintendent here.'

These ways of behaving with the patient were of course also helpful in protecting the relatives themselves from their own distress and uncertainty about the illness.

Discussion

The interviews which made up this study revealed a diversity of difficult experiences with some common threads. Many participants seemed to have a powerful need to tell their story and for several this was the first opportunity to do so. Often they found it difficult explicitly to express their own needs, although most were feeling overburdened by the situation.

An overwhelming feature of these interviews was that, despite the current philosophies of 'family-centred care', there was a lack of contact with health professionals. Nine of the participants had virtually no contact at all and for several others it had been minimal. Others described being 'in the dark', or 'in the wilderness'. However there was a certain ambivalence running through the relatives' interviews about help from professional carers. Many told me that they would not want any outsider to help provide care which they saw as their personal responsibility. This is illustrated by one woman who, when asked by the community nurse if she was coping with her husband's illness, said 'yes' because she was terrified that if she said 'no' her husband would be taken from her care. The nurse took this at face value and did not return for several weeks.

The variety of relationships and reactions to cancer exhibited in this study do not conform to a neat model. Perhaps it is the very diversity of the relationships, the reactions to the disease and the other things happening in the lives of the families which make them so difficult to assess and care for. However, there is evidence elsewhere in this study that support from nurses can reduce the additional worries and make the illness easier to bear, for example by giving information about treatment, or by ringing the family at home to see how they are getting on. The participants hoped that by telling their stories this would provide a better understanding, and that care for others would improve (although I myself was not always certain!). As with other research, it is the gap between what we know and think we *should* do and what we *actually* do, or have time to do, which is the crucial issue.

Acknowledgements

I would like to thank all those who took part in this study, my supervisor Alan Cribb for the discussions about this chapter and Cancer Relief Macmillan Fund for their support for this research.

References

Ball S J (1990) Self-doubt and soft data: Social and technical trajectories in ethnographic fieldwork. *Qualitative Studies in Education* 3(2):157–71.

Bliss J and Johnson B (1993) *Cancer patients' perceptions of need: Final Report.* London: Cancer Relief Macmillan Fund.

Bury M (1991) The sociology of chronic illness: A review of research and prospects. *Sociology of Health and Illness* 13(4):451–68.

Carey P J, Oberst M T, McCubbin M A and Hughs S H (1991) Appraisal and caregiving burden in family members caring for patients receiving chemotherapy. *Oncology Nursing Forum* 18(8):1341–8.

Cassileth B R and Hamilton J N (1979) The Family with Cancer. In: Cassileth B R (edn). *The Cancer Patient: Social and Medical Aspects of Care.* Philadelphia: Lea and Febiger.

Cornwell J (1984) *Hard-earned Lives: Accounts of Health and Illness from East London.* London: Tavistock Publications.

Cowles K V (1988) Issues in qualitative research on sensitive topics. *Western Journal of Nursing Research* **10**(2):163–79.

Daly K (1992) The Fit Between Qualitative Research and Characteristics of Families. In: Gilgun J, Daly K and Handel G (eds) *Qualitative Methods in Family Research*. London: Sage.

Darbyshire P (1994) Parenting in Public: Parental Participation and Involvement in the Care of their Hospitalised Child. In: Benner P (ed) *Interpretative Phenomenology*. London: Sage.

Ell K, Nishimoto R, Mantell J and Hamovitch M (1988) Longitudinal Analysis of Psychological Adaptation among Family Members of Patients with Cancer. *Journal of Psychosomatic Research* **32**(4/5):429–38.

Garrow L (1992) Chronic Illness and the Construction of Narrative. In: Del Vecchio Good M, Brodwin P, Good B and Kleinman A (eds) *Pain as Human Experience: An Anthropological Perspective*. Berkeley: University of California Press.

Given B, Dwyer T, Vredevoogd J and Given B (1988) Family Caregivers of Cancer: Reactions and Assistance. In: Pritchard P (ed) *Proceedings of the Fifth International Conference on Cancer Nursing*. London: Macmillan.

Glaser BD and Strauss AL (1967) *The Discovery of Grounded Theory*. New York: Aldine.

Hicks C (1988) *Who Cares: Looking After People at Home*. London: Virago Press.

Laslett B and Rapoport R (1975) Collaborative interviewing and interactive research. *Journal of Marriage and the Family* **37**:968–77.

Northouse L (1984) The Impact of Cancer on the Family: An Overview. *International Journal of Psychiatry in Medicine* **14**(3):215–42.

Oakley A (1981) Interviewing Women: A Contradiction in Terms. In: Roberts H (ed) *Doing Feminist Research*. London: Routledge and Kegan Paul.

Oberst M T and James R H (1985) Going home: patient and spouse adjustment following cancer surgery. *Topics in Clinical Nursing* **7**(1):46–57.

Plant H (1992) The Experiences of Relatives and Friends of Cancer Patients in the First Year after Diagnosis. In: Bailey C (ed) *Proceedings of the Seventh International Conference on Cancer Nursing*. Oxford: Rapid Communications.

De Raeve L (1992) Ethical issues in palliative nursing research: A question of kind? A question of degree? In: Bailey C (ed) *Proceedings of the Seventh International Conference on Cancer Nursing*. Oxford: Rapid Communications.

Reissman F (1976) How does self help work? *Social Policy* **7**(2):41–5.

RCN Standards of Care Project (1991) *Standards of Care for Cancer Nursing*. London: Royal College of Nursing.

Rolland J (1989) Chronic illness and the Family Life Cycle. In: Carter B and McGoldrick M (eds) *The Changing Family Life Cycle*. Boston: Allyn and Bacon.

La Rossa R, Bennett L A and Gelles R J (1981) Ethical dilemmas in qualitative family research. *Journal of Marriage and the Family* **43**:303–13.

Sales E (1992) Psychosocial Impact of the Phase of Cancer on the Family: An Updated Review. *Journal of Psychosocial Oncology* **9**(4):1–18.

Smith L (1992) Ethical Issues in Interviewing. *Journal of Advanced Nursing* **17**:98–103.

Del Vecchio Good M, Munakata T, Kobayashi Y, Mattingly C and Good B (1994) Oncology and Narrative Time. *Social Science and Medicine* **388**(6):855–62.

Webb C (1984) Feminist methodology in nursing research. *Journal of Advanced Nursing* **9**:249–56.

Chapter 9
Nurses and Involvement in Palliative Care Work
Katherine Froggatt

Introduction

This research study arose out of managerial concern in hospices for nurse employees who experienced personal bereavements whilst working with ongoing death and bereavement within their work environment. How do nurses cope with such events and what is the interaction between these two different types of loss – professional bereavement at work and personal loss at home?

In order to understand the impact of these events in nurses' lives it is first helpful to gain an insight into the nature of palliative care work. The relationships nurses develop with patients and families within the hospice are crucial for the delivery of high-quality, sensitive care. Involvement is a feature of these relationships between nurses and patients. Where involvement in relationships is facilitated by the hospice, it is more difficult to separate the professional and personal aspects of nurses' lives. The implications of involvement within palliative care work are considered in this chapter with reference to encounters with death and dying, both professional and personal.

Background Literature

The relationship between an individual's professional and personal life is considered by Vachon (1987). She has developed a 'Person-Environment Fit Model of Occupational Stress' that explicates the interaction between work and personal life. In her model the environmental (work) and personal aspects are present both as stressors and coping strategies. One specific area of stress discussed concerns working with dying and bereaved clients. However, the literature reveals a paucity of work that specifically considers the experience of multiple bereavements. The only consideration multiple losses receive is when they are mentioned as one of many stress factors for those who work in hospices (Vachon, 1978; Mount and Voyer, 1982; Yancik, 1984; Ray *et al*, 1987; Vachon, 1987; Taylor 1990). Within palliative care there is an understanding that bereavements are significant life events and this is recognised within hospices in the generally accepted practice, although no written guidelines exist, that staff will not be employed if they have undergone a personal bereavement in the previous year (Roche, 1981; Cooper, 1986). No formal provision is made for staff already working in a hospice who experience a personal bereavement.

A more general consideration of the bereavement literature indicates a widespread acceptance of a particular conceptual model. Teel (1991) in a review of the bereavement literature identifies this model as being temporally bound and linear, concerned with stages and process, as, for example, seen in the work by Lindemann (1944), Freud (1957), Parkes (1972) and Bowlby (1980). These staged linear models of bereavement are based on the assumption that each bereavement is a discrete event and an individual's response to that event follows a specific course. This model lacks flexibility in cases of chronic sorrow (Teel, 1991) or in situations where there are multiple or consecutive deaths.

Anthropological research demonstrates that Western society has clear life and death boundaries, with respect to space, time, medical control, social control and language (Hockey, 1990). The philosophy of the hospice movement blurs these boundaries in offering an alternative approach to prevailing medical ideals of cure and/or prevention (Abel, 1986). For example, hospice deaths are managed in an open and participatory way, rather than denied or hidden, as is more usual in acute hospital care. The experience of being in the nursing profession also informs nurses working within palliative care with respect to how they relate to patients and their families. There may be a conflict between their training as nurses and the approach to care as delivered within the hospice, especially with respect to the care of dying people. Nurses training within the hospital environment are constantly exposed to a medical approach to death, which is generally not based on the same premise as is a hospice approach. It has been suggested that dissatisfaction with the medical understanding of death may have been a reason why people move into palliative care (Vachon, 1987). Thus a hospice nurse is exposed to different views of care and death as a result of working within palliative care. Contradictory experiences may be encountered as the nurse tries to integrate the culture of the work environment and the social culture he/she lives in. To experience a death outside work may find the bereaved nurse having to integrate different understandings of death and dying.

Given these considerations this project, therefore, proposes to explore the interface between the professional and personal management and experience of death in Western society. The study is set in the cultural context of both the hospice and wider society. Attention is given to the specific ways in which death, dying and bereavement are managed by the hospice as an institution in which the nurse works, and the ways in which the nurse working within that institution experiences professional and personal losses. Regard is paid to the social, institutional and personal rituals which structure death, dying and bereavement. These may act as both stressors and supports to individuals.

Design and Methods

This qualitative research project uses a reflexive ethnographic approach to explore the aims outlined above. This involves situating the research within its cultural context which provides a rich ground for the exploration of the issues of death, dying and bereavement. By using ethnography the researcher attempts to understand what knowledge people use to interpret their experiences within the context of their culturally-defined environment (Aamodt, 1991). Reflexivity is the recognition that as a social researcher I am part of the social world I am investigating, and that there is an indivisibility of the subject and the object (Hammersley and Atkinson, 1983; Hockey, 1990). The focus of social interaction is the ethnographic interview and both participants, the nurses and myself as the researcher, create a relationship for the duration of the interview. The nature of this relationship can vary (Finch, 1984; Cannon, 1989) and this influences what the participants disclose of their experiences, and how they choose to do this. Rich data are obtained in the form of both information and perspective concerning the issues under consideration, (Hammersley and Atkinson, 1983). For example, interviews with nurses working in a particular hospice give very different accounts of the similar encounters with death within that environment, reflecting their own positions and experiences within that organisation.

Informal observation of the hospice culture occurred through ongoing observation in subsequent visits to the hospices. A further source of knowledge about the hospice culture is obtained from the literature produced by the hospices about themselves which is given to patients and their families. Throughout the study a reflective journal was kept by myself in which observations pertaining to the development of the research were noted. The use of supervision to discuss the interviews was also a part of the process of reflection.

The study involved taped in-depth interviews with female nurses (qualified and auxiliary) and their managers from four hospices located throughout England (table 9.1). The four hospices participating in the study cover the spectrum of hospices within England, in terms of their age, funding body and geography. Thirty-one interviews were with nurses from the four participating hospices and one interview was with a nurse who worked elsewhere and was willing to contribute. Six interviews were with nurse-managers in the hospices. Access to the hospice managers was obtained through professional contacts. After discussion with the nurse management in the hospices and ethical clearance from the relevant body, a letter was sent to all the nurses working in each hospice outlining details of the study and inviting their participation.

Table 9.1   Hospices and nurses participating in study

Hospice	No. of Beds*	Funding	Location	Managers	Qualified Nurses	Auxiliary Nurses
A	26	Independent	South East England	2	11	3
B	30	Independent	South East England	2	8	0
C	22	Charity	North England	1	6	1
D	20	NHS	South England	1	3	0

*Data from Hospice Information Service (1993)

Managers were interviewed using a semi-structured schedule to obtain information concerning the institutional management of professional and personal bereavements amongst its staff. In-depth interviews with bereaved nurses simultaneously explored the influence of personal loss on working with dying patients, and the experience of multiple work deaths on personal losses. The nurses were interviewed using a reflective story-telling approach (Graham, 1984; Schon, 1991). The interviews produced accounts of the management of, and experience of death, dying and bereavement from diverse viewpoints. The nurses being interviewed were asked to fulfil two criteria – that they had been in post for at least one year, and had experienced a personal bereavement of a significant person, at least six months ago. However, nurses who had experienced a personal loss but did not fulfil the above criteria were also included in the study if they felt they had something they wished to contribute.

Several ethical concerns were present throughout the research, not least the nature of the topic. This has affected the recruitment of the nurses into the study, how the interviews have been carried out, and the impact of undertaking such interviews for both the participant nurses and myself as the researcher. Careful consideration was given to these concerns by the researcher, particularly with respect to appropriate support for the nurses participating and for the researcher.

The analysis of the interview transcripts is currently being carried out using a constant comparative method. This arose as an integral part of the generation of grounded theory (Glaser and Strauss, 1967). Although this study is not attempting to develop theory, the principles of comparative content analysis to develop categories and themes provide a systematic way to analyse these data.

Findings and Discussion

In order to explore the experience of personal loss for nurses working within the palliative care specialty it is important to have an understanding of the nature of palliative care work. The findings presented in this chapter focus on this by exploring the relationship between nurses and the patients and families they care for. This relationship is shaped not only by the training nurses receive, but also by the environment within which they currently work.

Involvement is a recurring theme that underpins much of the nurses' discussion of their work in a hospice – a concept, it is argued, which is derived in part from the hospice culture. However, the personal losses experienced by the nurse may create different kinds of involvement. Distinctions can be drawn between institutional and interpersonal involvement. May (1991) differentiates between involvement as a general quality of nursing practice, and involvement as a personal attachment to specific patients. Involvement is structured by the hospice as an institution and within that context interpersonal involvement occurs between the nurses and the patients. Institutional involvement is manifested within the hospice as the organisational culture and ideology which shapes care practices, whereas interpersonal involvement occurs for nurses who have particular connections with specific patients. These distinctions are elaborated below.

Institutional Involvement

The structural aspects of involvement arise from the central organising philosophy of the hospice movement, an ideology which influences the palliative care given by nurses within specific hospices. From the examination of the symbolic language present in the literature given to patients and relatives from 125 English hospices, four hospice ideals which directly influence nurse–patient involvement are seen to be present:

- hospice as family;
- knowing the patients and families;
- an holistic approach to care;
- time for care.

These themes are interlinked and together they provide a coherent approach to the care a hospice provides for its patients, their family and friends. That these ideals are institutional is further illustrated by discussion of these same themes during the interviews with the nurses.

Hospice as Family
The idea of the hospice as family is an underlying feature of institutional involvement

and is depicted in the hospice literature. The hospice is represented as a family in the following excerpt from hospice literature:

> A hospice environment resembles a family, with the patient regarded as the much loved member of the family who has come to stay with his/her adoptive parents, the hospice team members providing the extended family figures. Family life as we are all well aware, is not all harmony; periods of discontent do occur. But with the commitment of the team to good internal and outside communication, the primary aim of ——— Hospice 'to serve the needs of the dying and their families' will be achieved.

The images presented here and elsewhere in hospice literature are partial and selective; the hospice does not always promote the negative aspects of family life, the tensions and disagreements. Rather it stresses the positive ideals. Even in the excerpt above, where discord is acknowledged, it is discussed in terms of the staff and their relationships rather than staff–client relationships. The staff are defined as the adults, making the patients figurative children. As symbolic dependants they therefore are not expected to be part of the 'adult' disputes.

Family life brings with it obligations and all members are required to take an active role within that setting. For staff therefore, involvement with patients, and close working relationships with all members of the multidisciplinary team, is part of being a member of the hospice family. The understanding conveyed by this imagery of the hospice as family is that here is a safe place with respect to relationships; people are close to each other, know and support each other. It also has implications for how the care is delivered, as this nurse describes:

> 'And I always try and think of the person that I'm looking after as a member of my family, and whether it be a man, or granddad, or mum, or a sister, how I would want them to be nursed.'

Knowledge
In order for the hospice to be a family the members need knowledge of each other, just as family members and close friends know each other. Davies and Oberle (1990) identify six dimensions of the supportive role of the nurse in palliative care. One of these is termed 'connecting' and concerns the nurse getting in touch with the patient and family; knowledge of the patient and family is an important aspect of this process. May (1991) similarly identifies knowledge and the need for reciprocity of knowledge as features of involvement between nurses and patients.

Knowledge of the patient by the nurse is integral to the creation of a relationship and it is through possessing knowledge of the patient that care is focused to meet any particular patient's needs. A nurse describes this process:

> 'Getting to know them as a patient, getting to know their fears, their problems,

anxieties, sharing, being able to listen and just to take time with them and their interests. I suppose being a friend to them. It's sort of being able to pick up when things aren't right with them. I mean once you do get to know them as a person then sort of more observant, if you like, of when there is a problem, you know it's not a personal, it's a real relationship, sort of when you are genuinely keeping an eye on them. Making sure things are going OK, being there when they need to cry or talk.'

The reason for getting to know a patient within a professional context is to create a relationship. 'Knowing the patient' gives the nurse a baseline from which to be able to identify when the situation changes for a patient. Relationships are necessary for good care to be provided for a patient. As the nurse above describes, this relationship may take different forms over time, 'being a friend' or having a 'real relationship', and this reflects the individual nurses and patients within any particular encounter. However, within a family and between close friends knowledge is mutual. If a hospice seeks to be a family and therefore implicitly affirms this particular type of relationship, nurses may be expected to reciprocate with knowledge about themselves, so transgressing their professional–personal boundary. The implications of reciprocity within nurse–patient relationships are explored further in the discussion around interpersonal involvement. Knowledge is not confined to knowing about someone as one just knows a friend, but also embraces the wider aspects of the person as espoused within holism.

Holism
The hospice movement places great emphasis on an holistic approach to care which views the individual as a whole, rather than as separate physical, emotional, social or spiritual parts. An excerpt from one hospice's patient booklet illustrates this:

The objectives for each caring member of the hospice movement are:
• to relieve distressing symptoms, such as pain, nausea etc by effective medication;
• to establish relaxed and easy communication with the patient in order to help dispel loneliness and to give opportunity for discussing the implications of his condition;
• to provide social, emotional, psychological and spiritual support in accordance with the needs of the patient and his family.

Here the physical needs of an individual are described as being met along with their social, psychological and spiritual needs, and the role the multidisciplinary team plays is depicted. By contrast, within a hospital context these aspects of a person are often divided between the medical staff, the family, the social worker and the church. The hospice promotes the fact that staff members are able to meet all needs. An important aspect of providing holistic care is physical contact. This ranges from the abstract concept of 'being there' to very close physical contact such as hugging or cuddling. Mediating between these extremes is the use of touch, as this nurse describes:

'I think touching is terribly important. You know, even if a person doesn't always respond, I think if you can just put an arm around somebody or just hold their hand, it's so important. And they do teach you to do that at this hospice.'

Many aspects of physical care, for example washing or toileting, require the nurse to be in close physical contact with the patient, an aspect of 'basic nursing care' increasingly missing in the high technology areas of hospital care. Indeed this aspect of hospice nursing work attracted some of the nurses interviewed to this area of nursing care. One feature of the emphasis on holistic care has been the increasing use of complementary therapies which also provide a vehicle for closeness. For example, massage is a form of therapy which requires touch between people. Physical contact becomes a medium for getting to know individuals, and through such contact personal space is transgressed, causing a breakdown of boundaries between self and other. This encourages social intimacy, creating the potential for greater closer interaction on other levels, for both the patient and the nurse.

However, holistic care is not only for the patient. An holistic approach means that the patient is not considered in isolation from the wider social context of family and friends, and care is extended to them as well. Moreover care is not confined to the period of time when the patient is alive, but continues to be offered to the relatives following the death of their family member in the form of bereavement follow-up and support:

The Hospice always has a positive approach to all problems so that it can help patients to live until they die and the family to go on living afterwards.

Holism in hospice nursing is therefore about unifying fragmented aspects of patient care. If this concept is applied to those practitioners offering holistic care, the implication is that there would be no separation, no boundary separating the professional and personal lives of the nurses.

Time
The final aspect of institutional involvement that hospices actively promote is the availability of time for patients and their families. Time is also identified by Ramos (1992) and Davies and Oberle (1990) as being necessary for close nurse–patient professional relationships. Ramos (1992) identifies that time was an important factor in the creation of relationships; she suggests that knowing the patient for shorter periods of time means it is more difficult to move to a deeper level of involvement.

Over time, often over a period of weeks and months, staff can establish relationships with their patients. One nurse describes how this occurs:

'Because you know your patients so well, this is the trouble. And some of them stay with us for such a long time.'

Within this passage of time there is also time available within the daily work, to be with patients and therefore to get to know them. That time is different in hospices from other health care settings is described by one nurse:

'You know you actually had time to ask a patient a question and listen to the answer. You didn't say, "Are you all right?" and keep on running, you know.'

Time is also necessary for physical contact to occur in any meaningful way, for it is often the time spent with a patient undertaking basic physical care which creates the context for getting to know the patient as a person. When time is present in both these ways the hospice ideals are met, as summarised in this hospice leaflet:

The staff take pride in welcoming you and hope that whilst with us you may feel part of our family. The team of nurses and doctors is backed up by social workers, chaplains and many volunteers who give freely of their time as good neighbours of the Hospice.
The gift of TIME is perhaps the one most important feature of Hospice Care – time to listen, time to care, to comfort, to concentrate on the needs and preferences of each individual patient. The staff are here to help you – don't hesitate to ask for their assistance on any matter worrying you.

By literally embodying involvement within palliative care work, as described above, hospices have created a particular environment within which their staff work through the facilitation of institutional involvement. These ideals affect both nurses' involvement in, and the nature of, relationships with patients and their families, relationships which may or may not lead to interpersonal involvement.

Interpersonal Involvement

As outlined earlier, involvement occurs when the professional and personal worlds of the nurse enter into each other. But interpersonal involvement does not occur in all nurse–patient relationships; instead, this kind of involvement is manifest between nurses and specific patients and their families. This may be either when the professional enters the personal, or when the personal enters the professional. The following extracts elucidate these two movements.

One nurse describes how professional issues enter her personal life:

'I don't really get sad about it at all, I go out and I can forget about it most of the time, might be one particular patient that really really got too, too close and will give me a disturbed night, or a bad week even, but on the whole I keep them fairly separate.'

In contrast another nurse recounts personal experience entering her professional world:

'Well, I just found that I understood how they felt, because as I said, I had lost so many of my family with cancer, and I just felt that I could put myself in their place and understand how they felt.'

The evidence from the interviews suggest that identification is a key factor in whether or not either form of interpersonal involvement occurs. Identification occurs when a connection is established between two individuals, as this nurse suggests:

'So, if it was somebody your own sort of age, with your own type of family, or that you just click, there are some patients you do . . . have a sort of rapport with, and they can be quite difficult, but you know when you meet them.'

Particular factors seem to shape whether such identification occurs. The nurses gave examples of identification with the disease of a patient, with their age, gender or common attributes. This identification is not always with self, but may be extended to either a family member who has died, or a live member of the family. One nurse talks about her identification with a patient because of similarities with her live son and other shared experiences.

'. . . and he had such a wicked sense of humour that I think his sense of humour was on a par with my son's and maybe that was something that made it special, I don't know. We had a lot of interests in common as well. He was a great one for going to T——— and that's one of my favourite spots, and just various things that we had, a great deal in common . . .'

Problems may be encountered when nurses identify with patients. In the following account, a nurse describes an incident where she was not able to stay with a patient:

'The son was dying. I think in his 30s, and she had a lot of children, but he was her favourite. Now I've got one son and I don't know what on earth possessed me, I don't reverse roles like that. But I thought, "What if that's my son there?" And I've never done that before – never, and I just thought, "Oh my God, I wish somebody would come." I said, "No, I'm gonna have to go."'

And at that point the nurse had to leave the patient. Through identification this nurse was experiencing a breakdown of her family boundaries as she imagined the loss of her own son. The result of such an episode is a nurse who is unable to continue to give care to that particular patient and family.

That nurses identify with patients even when their professional and personal boundaries are well maintained has implications for nurses who have experienced a personal bereavement. Their being already more vulnerable emotionally and in a state of transition may affect their ability to maintain their personal and professional boundaries. A 'rites of passage' model, drawn from anthropology, offers an alternative way to understanding bereavement. The bereaved individual is in a transitory, liminal state (Van Gennep, 1960), neither in the pre-bereavement state, nor in the position of having resolved their grief, and is thus left in an ambiguous situation. One consequence of occupying this transitory state that a bereaved nurse may encounter is identification with the patients she cares for, particularly with respect to the person who has died, as this nurse describes:

'But it affects me now, in as much as when I see a man with gastric cancer I can see my father.'

This type of personal identification with the death of someone close to the nurse can have a direct impact on the nurse's ability to care for particular patients. Another nurse describes the times she is not able to care for people:

'. . . 'cause I can't nurse people who've got colon with liver secondaries – not at the end. On a good day I can, but the staff are aware that if I say "No, I can't sit with somebody", they don't question it. They just say "OK, somebody else will do it." But on a, when I'm going through one of my bad times, I can't, 'cause it's just like seeing my husband dead.'

It should be noted that the nurses also described how they use their identification through personal experience as a means to become closer to patients, as this nurse recounts:

'And I think it's been more helpful than – I mean obviously my own sadness and loss I've had to cope with, but it's another dimension that I've, has been placed upon me and I hope that I've learned from it and made some sense of it, and I think, I think, I don't know, perhaps it gives me an added empathy and perhaps that sounds very arrogant but I don't know.'

Within the context of professional relationships between nurses and patients, nurses may find that identification draws on their personal life and experiences. Morse (1991) suggests that nurses may use an establishment of common ground to develop involvement with a patient. This is an active use of identification to negotiate a relationship which will then be beneficial to the patient.

Bereaved nurses may find themselves in a position to identify more closely with patients and families, because of their own experiences. This may have negative effects on their work, but over time individuals may be enabled to use these experiences positively to enhance their relationships with patients.

Conclusion

Involvement is a feature of palliative care work as delivered by hospices. The hospice facilitates an environment of structured involvement between nurses and patients. When faced with death, patients and their families may be particularly vulnerable and find it difficult to allow strangers close to them. In order to develop holistic 'family' relationships, nurses may find themselves sharing personal knowledge in order to gain the confidence of patients. The length and intensity of time which nurses know patients further adds to the involvement present in these relationships.

Identification does occur between nurses and their patients, and this can be beneficial for nurse–patient relationships. That involvement and identification occurs in the course of nursing care has implications for nurse-managers and the nurses themselves. Nurse-managers are expected to provide support for their nursing staff that allows them to continue to work professionally and compassionately with patients and their families. This support needs to enhance the individual nurse's maintenance of his/her professional and personal boundaries. Nurses need to develop an awareness of their own work which will allow them to know when they are identifying and becoming involved with patients in a way which is not beneficial for either themselves or the patient.

When nurses experience personal events outside work, their ability to maintain their boundaries between their professional and personal lives may be compromised. This leads to the nurses being more vulnerable in the work situation, and they may then be more likely to identify in a way which is not beneficial for their work. An understanding that this may occur means that managers need to know their staff so as to be able to perceive when particular relationships between nurses and patients are detrimental to either party.

The issues discussed here also need to be put into the context of the larger study from which this discussion on involvement is derived. This project originated from a concern expressed by hospice managers regarding the experience of personal bereavement of their employees. The interviews with the nurses are also exploring their experience of death, dying and bereavement both professionally and personally. The findings presented here begin to shed light on some of the implications for nurses' work of encounters with professional and personal bereavement. Further analysis of this data will explore the ways nurses manage their work following personal bereavements.

Acknowledgements

Thanks are due to Allison James and Judy Allsop, without whom this study would not have come so far.

The findings presented here are part of an ongoing doctoral study undertaken at South Bank University.

References

Aamodt A M (1991) Ethnography and Epistemology: Generating Nursing Knowledge. In: Morse J M (ed) *Qualitative Nursing Research: A Contemporary Dialogue.* Newbury Park, California: Sage.

Abel E K (1986) The hospice movement: Institutionalizing innovation. *International Journal of Health Services* 16(1):71–85.

Bowlby J (1980) *Attachment and Loss:* Volume 3: *Loss, Sadness and Depression.* New York: Basic Books.

Cannon C (1989) Social research in stressful settings: Difficulties for the sociologist studying the treatment of breast cancer. *Sociology of Health and Illness* 11(1):62–77.

Cooper M (1986) Staff Selection. In: Turnball P (ed) *Terminal Care.* Washington: Hemisphere.

Davies B and Oberle K (1990) Dimensions of the supportive role of the nurse in palliative care. *Oncology Nursing Forum* 17(1):87–94.

Finch J (1984) 'It's great to have someone to talk to': the ethics and politics of interviewing women. In: Bell C and Roberts H (eds) *Social Researching: Politics, Problems, Practice.* London: Routledge and Kegan Paul.

Freud S (1957) Mourning and Melancholia. In: Strachey J (ed. and trans.) *Standard Edition of the Complete Psychological Works of Sigmund Freud.* London: Hogarth Press.

Van Gennep A (1960) *The Rites of Passage.* London: Routledge and Kegan Paul.

Glaser B D and Strauss A L (1967) *The Discovery of Grounded Theory.* New York: Aldine.

Graham H (1984) Surveying through stories. In: Bell C and Roberts H (eds) *Social Researching: Politics, Problems, Practice.* London: Routledge and Kegan Paul.

Hammersley M and Atkinson P (1983) *Ethnography: Principles in Practice.* London: Tavistock.

Hockey J (1990) *Experiences of Death.* Edinburgh: Edinburgh University Press.

Hospice Information Service (1993) *Directory of Hospice Services.* London: St Christopher's Hospice.

Lindemann E (1944) Symptomatology and management of acute grief. *American Journal of Psychiatry* **101**:141–8.

May C (1991) Affective neutrality and involvement in nurse–patient relationships: perceptions of appropriate behaviour among nurses in acute medical and surgical wards. *Journal of Advanced Nursing* **16**:552–8.

Morse J M (1991) Negotiating commitment and involvement in the nurse–patient relationship. *Journal of Advanced Nursing* **16**:455–68.

Mount B M and Voyer J (1982) Staff stress in palliative/hospice care. In: Ajemian I and Mount B M (eds) *The Royal Victoria Hospital Manual on Palliative/Hospice Care.* Salem: Ayer.

Parkes C M (1972) *Bereavement: Studies of Grief in Adult Life.* New York: International Universities Press.

Ramos M C (1992) The nurse–patient relationship: theme and variations. *Journal of Advanced Nursing* **17**:496–506.

Ray E B, Nichols M R and Perritt L J (1987) A model of job stress and burnout. *The Hospice Journal* **3**(2/3):3–28.

Roche K (1981) Staff selection, education and evaluation. In: Zimmerman J M (ed) *Hospice: Complete Care for the Terminally Ill.* Baltimore: Urban and Schwarzenberg.

Schon D A (1991) *The Reflective Practitioner.* London: Avebury.

Taylor J (1990) Coping with the stress on carers. *The Practitioner*, 22 March, **234**:300–1.

Teel C S (1991) Chronic sorrow: Analysis of the concept. *Journal of Advanced Nursing* **16**:1311–19.

Vachon M L S (1978) Motivation and stress experienced by staff working with the terminally ill. *Death Education* **2**:113–22.

Vachon M L S (1987) *Occupational Stress in the Care of the Critically Ill, the Dying, and the Bereaved.* New York: Hemisphere.

Yancik R (1984) Coping with hospice work stress. *Journal of Psychosocial Oncology* **2**(2):19–35.

Section Four

Emotional Reactions and Communication Issues

Chapter 10
Emotional Disclosure between Cancer Patients and Nurses
Anne Lanceley

Introduction

Cancer nurses accept that the expression of emotion and the disclosure of feelings may affect the cancer patient's ability to adjust to their diagnosis and cope with their treatment (McMahon and Pearson, 1991). They acknowledge, too, the power of communication in its capacity to provoke or ameliorate the fear that often accompanies cancer (Lichter, 1987; Ley, 1988).

Also a belief in the interdependence and unity of body and mind may not be a mere theoretical notion for cancer nurses but one they claim to experience in their daily practice (Del Vecchio Good *et al*, 1990). Recognition of this has perhaps distinguished cancer nursing and led to early critical concern over the nature, content and quality of the nurse–patient relationship in cancer-care settings (Morrow *et al*, 1976; Holmes, 1988; May, 1992).

Thus cancer nurses strive to embody what Benner confidently terms 'the helping role' (Benner, 1984). This involves:

- Finding an acceptable interpretive understanding of the illness, pain, fear, anxiety or other stressful emotion;
- Assisting the patient to use social, emotional or spiritual support;
- Mobilising hope for the nurse as well as the patient.

The potential of this 'therapeutic sensibility,' in cancer care is recognised across the health-care disciplines (Blum, 1985) but by none more so than nurses (Uys, 1980; Carpenter and Morrow, 1986; McMahon and Pearson, 1991). What is less certain is whether oncology nurses do, in practice, accept and deal with the emotions patients express to them. For, despite the increasing interest and rhetoric surrounding this subject, research studies to date suggest that nurses' communication with cancer patients remains superficial (Bond, 1978; Hunt, 1989; Wilkinson, 1991).

It is this apparent mismatch which fascinates me as an oncology nurse and educator and which is under investigation in the study described in this chapter.

Two aspects of emotional disclosure are explored in the study. First, how patients express their feelings to the nurses who care for them and what happens in the interaction when they do. Second, the implications and consequences to the nurse of the emotional disclosure.

What is Emotional Disclosure?

A discursive approach to emotions demands that emotion is neither regarded as a pure physiological experience nor simply describable in the terms of cognitive psychology, for it is also a matter of cultural and social construction. As Rosaldo suggests:

> Feelings are not substances to be discovered in our blood but social practices organised by stories that we both enact and tell. They are structured by our forms of understanding.
>
> (Rosaldo, 1984)

Cultural prescriptions and social norms thus become most important determinants of emotional display, disclosure and management (Hochschild, 1979; Kemper, 1981, Harre, 1986). Accordingly emotions cannot be understood outside their social context. A contextual approach is therefore adopted for this study.

Another important characteristic of emotion is that all knowledge or understanding of emotion is intersubjective and there is nothing intrinsic to a social context or situation which makes it, or the people in it, either 'emotional' or 'unemotional'. Thus any patient account, considered within the remit of this study to be emotionally disclosive, may be only speculatively so. This is further complicated by the fact that emotional disclosure is largely under voluntary control while emotional experience is not. A patient may be able to make themselves sound as though they accept their diagnosis but they cannot make themselves feel this. Therefore the emotions felt and the emotions described or shown by the patient may be poles apart (Hochschild, 1983). Emotional disclosure involves cancer patients in an essential human activity of first deciding whether to reveal their feelings or past emotional experiences to another. They must decide at what level of intimacy to reveal the personal information and the appropriate time, place and target person for the disclosure. Not surprisingly such disclosure is believed to have consequences for an individual's thoughts and feelings about 'self' (Derlaga and Berg, 1987).

Ideas of self add another important dimension to the concept of emotional disclosure. To a relatively new breed of 'discursive psychologists' (Potter and

Wetherell, 1987; Shotter and Gergen, 1992), talk is overtly functional. It is used to get things done. Emotional disclosure is therefore deemed to be one method available to individuals of 'making sense' of their experience. In turn 'methods of making sense' are the key to any explanation of the self. Clearly this new breed of social psychologist subscribes to a 'social constructionist' idea of the self whereby there is not one fixed self waiting to be discovered but a multiplicity of selves found in the different kinds of linguistic practices articulated now and in the past (Gergen, 1985). Emotional disclosure is, therefore, a way cancer patients construct 'self'.

It is this distinctive view of the self and conversation which informs the choice of a discourse-analytic method for this study: a method which places the emphasis firmly on the talk, how it is constructed and how it functions. The research approach also owes much to previous work by Nik and Justine Coupland who examined painful self-disclosure as a characteristic of intergenerational talk (Coupland and Coupland, 1988). Their careful and detailed analysis, culminating in a taxonomic overview of the range of strategies interactants used to negotiate the exchange of intimate painful information, provided an early model for the conduct of the study.

Emotional Disclosure and Cancer

The idea that styles of emotional disclosure and, in particular, actively holding back from expressing feelings, may not only render a person 'cancer prone', but also affect the progress of the cancer illness, has been a powerful one in the cancer literature and perhaps in the minds of cancer patients for more than three decades (Doan and Gray, 1992).

There is a notion that cancer patients suffer from repressed deep-seated emotional traumata or conflicts, bound with negative emotions such as anger, frustration or guilt. Being repressed, these feelings constitute a chronic source of stress turned against the self and manifested somatically in cancer (LeShan and Worthington, 1956; Greer, 1983).

Most investigators assume, at least implicitly, that repression is characteristic of cancer patients and is somehow involved in the occurrence of cancer. In contrast Kreitler et al argue that repression is a response to the extreme stress posed by the cancer diagnosis. When faced with a threat to physical existence, an individual may be flooded with such intense anxiety that repression is a natural defence (Kreitler et al, 1993). Kreitler's work accords with the conclusions reached by Greer et al that denial, fighting spirit, stoic acceptance or helplessness/hopelessness are responses to cancer illness, and in this case they are state-specific and not indicative of a personality trait (Greer et al, 1979).

Work has also examined the relationship between emotional expression and the way cancer patients cope with their illness and its ramifications. More emotionally distressed patients were found to use passive, submissive and suppressive coping strategies while patients with lower distress tended to confront problems directly, seek solutions, get information and share their concerns (Weisman and Worden, 1977).

Emotional Disclosure in the World of Cancer Care

Glaser and Strauss were the first to begin to expose the profound emotional basis for the social organisation and context of care in relation to cancer patients and the dying. In their important study of disclosure they not only identified the troubling reality of awareness categories, but also described ways in which knowledge about diagnosis and prognosis was used to disallow or control emotions (Glaser and Strauss, 1965).

James develops this theme of emotion management in her examination of the disclosure of a cancer diagnosis. She describes the management of own and others' emotions at this time by lay and professional carers, noting that many manage by denying rather than engaging with emotions (James, 1993). Differences in emotion management she attributes to different levels of involvement with the feelings associated with the cancer and competing forms of status and knowledge. These then influence the mechanisms used to manage the feelings such as the use of particular kinds of space and time, more or less public encounters, denial of the emotion, limiting the information released, formal and informal disciplinary rules, gender-divided labour and, most significantly, senior staff setting the context, routines and rituals within which other staff and clients can express their feelings.

An interesting examination of the emotionally charged moral activity of representing hopefulness on a leukaemic ward similarly revealed that interactional 'Hope Work' is conducted within a medical frame and serves the purpose of maintaining the legitimacy and credibility of the medical version of reality (Perakyla, 1991).

The findings from these studies suggest that feelings contribute to and reflect the structure and culture of the cancer-care setting. It is useful to consider cancer specific nurse–patient interaction studies in this light.

In an early study Quint observed that nurses denied the reality of cancer and possible death not only to avoid negative reactions but to further hope in the face of uncertainty (Quint, 1965).

Holmes and Dickerson indicated that cancer patients felt unable to discuss their anxieties with nursing staff, perceiving them to be too busy and too young to understand the implications of a cancer diagnosis (Holmes and Dickerson, 1987).

Bond reported that during her study nurses believed that open discussion by patients of their feelings concerning the possible consequences of their illness would do more harm than good, that it would prompt displays of excessive emotion and that patients would become hysterical, cry or withdraw, becoming morbid or even suicidal. Nurses perceived patients as simply giving up all hope in these circumstances (Bond, 1978).

Maguire found that nurses tended to ignore signs of distress from patients, instead of allowing patients to lead the conversation and talk about their worries. Nurses did not engage with patients or if they did, spoke in clichés. There was little acknowledgement of the uniqueness of each patient's coping style or a recognition of the patient's need to be nurtured and affirmed through communication (Maguire, 1985).

It is hard to contemplate that nurses today would maintain such a view and ignore obvious verbal and non-verbal cues exhibited by patients who are distressed. Yet nurses, it appears, use a variety of tactics, whether consciously or not, to avoid communicating at anything but a superficial level.

In an ethnomethodological case study of a single patient's 'career as a breast cancer patient', Tait draws attention to ways in which she organised her talk with her patient; how she controlled conversation and established it on her own terms (Tait, 1986). One way this was managed was by contributing words to the patient's talk. The example given concerns how the patient related to her husband after her mastectomy.

Pt. It builds a barrier, I think.
N. Yes.
Pt. Erm . . .
N. Can you just say how you feel – is it that you feel incomplete?
Pt. Yes.
N. I think that was the word you said, wasn't it?
Pt. Well erm . . . I can't really say – really – you feel so erm . . . abnormal.
N. Yes, Yes.

The recognition that nurses are failing to respond and help patients and their families express their fears and feelings about cancer, death, pain and loss stimulated an influential study (Wilkinson, 1991). Wilkinson adapted Forrest's scale of 'blocking' or 'facilitating' behaviours to rate tape-recorded nursing history-taking (Forrest, 1983). Wilkinson examined this process with regard to newly diagnosed patients with cancer, patients who had developed a recurrence and patients admitted for palliative care.

Wilkinson found 54 per cent of verbal behaviours to be 'blocking' and the patients who occasioned the most 'blocking' behaviours were those returning to hospital with a recurrence of disease. A further dimension of the study was multiple-regression analysis of predictor variables for those nurses who 'facilitated' and for those who 'blocked'. The ward in which the nurse worked was found to be a significant predictor for both 'facilitators' and 'blockers'. Wards in which there was an 'open awareness' context resulted in a much higher proportion of 'facilitating' behaviours. High 'blocking' behaviours were influenced by the ward and in particular the ward sister's manner and distancing from her patients.

Hunt reports similar minimal emotional disclosure between dying patients, their families and symptom control nurses in the community. For, she argues, patients and relatives 'adapted to deal with emotionally charged situations' by 'ordinary behaviour'. Consequently, nurses largely ignored existential worries of patients. Conversational processes which promoted expression of feelings were very limited (Hunt, 1989).

The Nurse, the Patient and Emotional Disclosure: Evidence from this Study

The first aim of the study was to identify emotional material in talk between nurses and cancer patients and to explore the processes by which this material was managed.

Consequently, the first data set consisted of 60 nurse–patient interactions tape-recorded in hospital oncology units and patients' homes during follow-up care. The 23 participating oncology-trained nurses initiated the tape-recording during the course of their day-to-day nursing activities and interaction with patients.

The data were transcribed and subjected to detailed discourse analysis. This textual analysis consisted of identifying categories of notionally painful topics. These were:

- Physiological effects of illness or treatment;
- Change in lifestyle, accustomed habits and activities due to illness;
- Effect on family and friends, those at home;
- Why me? Searching for meaning;
- Response to current state of ill-health or situation;
- Other life issues, e.g. divorce, single parenthood, bereavement, plight of another patient.

The next stage in the analysis was to focus on the emotionally disclosive sequences within the conversations. Disclosive sequences were found to consist of four phases. The range of alternative verbal strategies used by the nurses and patients during the phases of the emotional sequence was then analysed in detail.

Pre-contexts
This phase distinguishes three broad means by which subsequent disclosures are triggered:

- Nurse-determined (elicitation of emotional disclosure by nurse);
- Textually determined (where considerations of conversational coherence

predispose or require an emotional disclosure);
• Patient-determined (where the pre-context to make an emotional disclosure is established by the patient him/herself).

Ways of disclosing

These are characterised along various dimensions, including the thematic prominence afforded to the 'core' of an emotional disclosure within the conversation, and 'elaboration' – that is, the complexity of functional units comprising a disclosive sequence. Issues of prosody and paralinguistics are considered here. Though of obvious importance, the non-verbal accompaniment to a disclosure is not given prominence in this study.

Next moves of nurse to manage the disclosure

These fall into numerous minimal and full moves which variously enable or inhibit further emotional disclosure.

Moves of nurse or patient to close

These are defined as the first contributions in each of the emotionally disclosive sequences, made by either the patient or the nurse, towards closing the topic and stopping on-going emotional talk. (This is independent of whether or not, in the flow of talk, closure is actually achieved.)

The phases described assisted in structurally defining portions of conversation as units for analysis. Figure 10.1 represents them in summary form.

The use of short extracts will enrich this summary material, expose the analysis technique for scrutiny and in so doing offer insights into the very real difficulties of talking to cancer patients. A description of the transcription notation used in the extracts is to be found at the end of this chapter.

Extract 1

```
35 N. Have you seen your children recently
36 P. I see them often (slowly)
37 N. Do they come up in the evening
38 P. Yeh(.) I mean it does me good to have them here (1.6) my brother coming
39     they sort of cheer me up if anything • like I need like I'm (1.2) I don't feel
40     better • but I will go home for a break and come back and feel better (1.2)
41     but now      ⌈I feel like =
42                  ⌊Yes
43 N.
44 P. =A mega problem
45 N. Why do you feel that
```

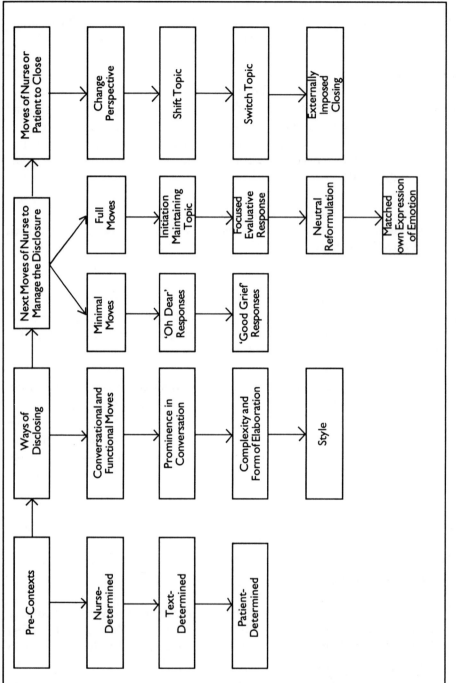

Figure 10.1 Phases within emotionally disclosive sequences
Summary of verbal strategies

46 P. I fe::el it in my body (quietly)
47 N. Do you uh
48 P. Mmm (1.6) I feel lousy today and all the time
49 N. Don't you feel any hope at the moment (gently)
50 P. I couldn't ca::re (sadly)
51 N. I mean you've been told your counts are getting better
     they   ⌈actually told =
52 P.   ⌊Mmm
53 N. = Told you that today • have they said when they want to give you more
    treatment

In the above extract the nurse asks the patient directly about her children. This is likely to elicit information within one of the emotional disclosure topic categories, given the long hospitalisation of this young woman with leukaemia. The patient responds and satisfies demands for textual coherence but elaborates and discloses further information concerning her feelings when her family visit. Also she discloses her feelings concerning her physical state. Though the nurse gives a focused evaluative response at 1.45 and engages in a 'full' conversational move to maintain the topic at 1.49 she subsequently denies the individual patient's perspective and does not pursue her risk-taking line of questioning concerning hope. The sequence is 'closed' when the nurse lightens the talk and effects a change of key by introducing positive clinical results to frame the patient's feelings of 'couldn't care'.

The above extract illustrates several important findings of the study. First, that emotional disclosure is a pervasive and overwhelming feature in all the interactions analysed irrespective of the nurse's response. Patients do behave disclosively and talk about the meaning of their illness and their own death. Further, though nurses demonstrate responsive communication skills, these are not consistently used even within a single conversation.

Analysis also reveals that the way in which emotion is disclosed and how it is managed is not an individual patient phenomenon nor wholly engineered and controlled by the nurse. Instead emotional disclosure emerges as a collaborative venture between the nurse and patient within the give and take of conversation.

Extracts 2 and 3 illustrate some further findings through analysis – in particular that patient's predominant mode of emotional expression is metaphoric and embodied. A young woman with ovarian cancer, looking in the mirror at herself, spoke to the nurse.

Extract 2

P. Oh look at me (1.6) look at my eyes (they were very sunken and dark)
N. Mmm

P. Like two holes in the sno::w

N. You don't look <u>that</u> bad

P. I feel it

The nurse in this extract appears to have difficulty inferring emotional experience from the patient's verbal behaviour since the patient did not use affect words or at first directly comment on her feelings. Another example was a lady with a recurrence of her breast cancer who likened her body to 'a piece of wood which someone keeps knocking nails into'. Her description was ignored by the nurse.

Extract 3 concerns a middle-aged woman with late-stage disease who throughout an hour-long conversation with a nurse, referred to herself as a 'fool'. She used a light bantering style of talk and described how her children spoke of her as being 'a laugh' and how even her doctor had commented that 'She didn't mind nothing, did she?' Towards the end of the conversation the woman speaks of a saving the children could make.

Extract 3

P. I told them they could all save their money Christmas (.) instead of buying me lots of little presents they can buy me a gun and I'll pop meself off (Laughs)

N. Is that what it makes you feel like sometimes (reflective)

P. Well (3.4) ye::h (.) I think you do::don't ya

N What would make you feel like that (.) if the pain got very bad or something (2.1) or just general sort of thinking about being unwell

P. I don't know

N. You don't know (1.2)

P. It's just my word (.) just er my joke really

N. Just your joke

P. Ye:::h

N Okay (.) Well listen if what you're planning to do is go home and get back to <u>normal</u> (0.8) let's aim for that shall we

The nurse, it could be said, ignores the patient's covert expression of feeling.

In summary the findings of this first data set represent two levels of emotional disclosure. At one level, the overt, conscious, surface level, there may be very few conversational 'next moves' open to the nurse which can be regarded as 'safe'. Children, friends, holidays and activities can all prove to be an emotional mine-field. The nurse is then engaged in the anxiety-provoking work of 'response-finding'.

At another level entirely the patient confronts and reflects the unbearableness of their situation *covertly* through word choice, prosody and extraordinarily powerful idiosyncratic, metaphoric and embodied language. During the emotionally disclosive, 'sense-making' sequences, the patients are essentially using their bodies to 'think' with.

This process can occur at a conscious level but also exists at a deep unconscious level, and as such is expressive of the profound emotional experience of having a life-threatening illness. The 'death head' metaphor for the ovarian cancer patient and the 'nails in the coffin' image described by the lady with recurrent illness, it is suggested, operate at this deep level.

Analysis of the second data set attempts to throw light upon these findings and illuminate the nurses' verbal behaviours. If, as evidenced here, oncology nurses do have the skills to meet the emotional needs of cancer patients why is the nurses' use of these patchy? Could it be that nurses are consciously or unconsciously blocking their skills?

Consequences of Patients' Emotional Disclosure on the Nurses

The approach to analysing this second data set was primarily informed by the experience of the interviews with the nurses. The nurses demonstrated an overwhelming orientation to their self-image and self-presentation in relation to their talk with patients.

The interview was a ground for self-disclosures concerning nurses' perceptions of their private and professional selves.

   N. I wonder if I should reveal so much of myself (to patients) and I think sometimes it doesn't matter

It appeared important for some nurses to describe their relationship and closeness to patients.

   N. This was a person (.) although this tape sounds really hard and it comes over like that this is a person who I since learnt really liked me and felt comfortable with me as a nurse

Most participants found the interview 'threatening' to some degree. This is perhaps not surprising since not only were the nurses presented with transcribed 'evidence' of their talk with patients during the interview, they were asked to account for their verbal strategies. Information was also sought on their thoughts and feelings at the time of their conversation with the patient. Essentially, therefore, the nurse subjects were engaged in a self-disclosive process during the interview with me.

Disclosure is a sensitive business and constitutes a 'face-threatening' situation to social psychologist Erwin Goffman. It is necessary to elaborate on this concept, for it emerged as a suitable path leading into analysis of the interview data.

Goffman (1955) defines 'face' as

The positive social value a person effectively claims for himself by the line others assume he has taken during a particular contact.

Consequently two broad classes of identity concerns motivate people – 'positive face', which is the desire to be well regarded and 'negative face', the desire not to be imposed upon.

These account for most instances of communication exchanges. In further work Goffman (1959) developed his theory to explain the routine ways people present themselves in everyday life: how they support or challenge others' 'face' claims and deal with challenges to their own 'face'. According to Goffman, we use various strategies to enhance, defend, protect, threaten or depreciate our negative and positive 'faces' all the time.

The interview data were examined for these self-presentational concerns in relation to the *overt* and *covert* ways in which patients expressed their feelings to the nurse. A complex dynamic of nurses 'face-work' and defensiveness emerged from analysis of the interview data (figure 10.2).

Complementing these findings was the fact that nurses openly acknowledge the difficulties of responding to patients' feelings. Nurses expressed worry about what in a particular instance would be therapeutic or beneficial to the patient. Concerns about their identity and image as a responsive, compassionate nurse who could deal confidently with their own feelings as well as those of the patient were frankly discussed during the interview.

From these data the amount of 'face-work' undertaken by the nurse subjects during the interview relates to their range of responsive talk with patients. Nurses who expressed minimal anxiety concerning participation in the study and who were less protective and defensive of their 'face' used significantly more responsive ways of talking with patients and were more likely to have noted the patients' covert modes of emotional expression at the time of conversation and to have acted upon this knowledge.

Discussion

The research reported here has focused on the content and process of emotional disclosure between oncology-trained nurses and their patients and the opinions and feelings of the nurses concerning these communications. The main findings and issues raised by the study are now addressed.

Face	To: Enhance	To: Defend/Protect	To: Threaten	To: Depreciate
POSITIVE (Desire to be well regarded)	• Express magnanimity • Say positive things about self	• Explain reasons for communication • Defend truthfulness of account • Defend appropriateness of communication • Seek sympathy	• Admit inappropriateness of communication • Concede • Give deference • Sardonic comments/jokes about self	• Self-accusation • Admit faults
NURSE SELF				
NEGATIVE (Avoidance of contempt for self)	• Assert rights • Refuse advice/direction	• Hedge cooperation • Give insufficient information • Give no direct response • Hedge commitment	• Accept advice/direction • Admit constraints • Accept obligation	• Relinquish control
		No direct Face-work Effect • Direct answer with extension	No direct Face-work Effect • Direct maximal efficient answer	

Figure 10.2 Face-work strategies during nurse-researcher interviews

Emotional Disclosure and Cancer

Overwhelmingly patients did disclose their feelings to nurses and did raise existential concerns, for emotional disclosure was a recurring but variable component of talk across the data base. This accords with literature describing the importance for patients of disclosing their feelings (Mitchell and Glicksman, 1977; Fiore, 1979; Cohen, 1981; Pistrang and Barker, 1992). The finding does, however, contrast with the work of Quint, McIntosh, Bond, Drummond-Mills, and Hunt, who all highlight the difficulties nurses find in talking to cancer patients and consequent low levels of emotional expression in conversation (Quint, 1965; McIntosh, 1974; Bond, 1978; Drummond-Mills, 1983; Hunt, 1989).

The collaborative nature of the disclosure episodes is a phenomenon not identified in previous studies of nurse-talk with cancer patients (Bond, 1978; Maguire, 1985; Wilkinson, 1991). These studies either were designed to gain a general picture of interaction in terms of amount of talk and range of topics or allowed only for the identification of nurses' verbal behaviours. The studies present a consistent picture of nurses 'blocking' or 'discouraging' patients from disclosing difficult or painful information. The chosen contextual, discourse-analytic method of analysis used in this study allows identification of the joint contributions of participants, thus offering insight into the day-to-day experience and difficulties of nurses talking with cancer patients.

When we turn to the way patients express their feelings, the higher proportion of covert to overt expression within the nurse–patient conversations supports empirical work in this field demonstrating that cancer patients are characterised by poor direct expression of emotions, especially negative ones like anger, depression and hostility (Cox and McKay, 1982; Greer and Watson, 1987; Bacon, 1988; Taylor *et al*, 1988).

In other studies cancer patients score high on covert anxiety and on alexithymia – that is an inability to describe their feelings (Schonfield, 1975; Todarello *et al*, 1989). This is reflected in the findings of this study that though patients did talk about their feelings they often relied on metaphoric, indirect models of disclosure.

The implications of this become clear when the evidence concerning the effect of repressing feelings is taken into account. An emotionally repressive style and low expression of negative affect has been directly related by some researchers to disease spread in cancer patients (Derogatis *et al*, 1979; Temshok, 1985; Jensen, 1987), while others claim that the effect of denial and repression of feelings may positively influence coping adjustment and thence survival (Weisman and Worden, 1975; Greer *et al* 1979; Lonnqvist, 1981; Cassileth, Lusk and Miller, 1985; Pettingale *et al*, 1985). If further research reveals negative effects of repression on survival and the quality of cancer patients' illness experience, then it is incumbent upon the nurse to respond to patients' overt and covert expressions of feelings.

The study raises interesting questions about the ways patients make sense of their experience and cope with the cancer illness. Sontag first gave prominence to the idea that metaphor plays a significant role in the construction of cancer illness. She argues eloquently that people with cancer are the subject of 'punitive and sentimental fantasies' concocted about them and their illness. Part of her thesis is that the generation of metaphor is not an innocent quest of random discovery or individual creativity but a purposeful method society has for controlling and conferring advantage or disadvantage and making moral judgements on those with cancer. The most truthful and, by implication, healthiest way of being ill with cancer is therefore one purified of metaphoric thinking (Sontag, 1978).

Evidence presented in this study suggests that we cannot strip metaphor away. On the contrary, patients in the study consistently use metaphor to give effective expression to the demands of their cancer illness, particularly in relation to matters of uncertainty, fear, pain and stigma.

Furthermore, there is evidence that patients used their bodies as a rich metaphoric source for the expression of their distress. This accords with recent work by psychotherapists and medical anthropologists alike, who claim that to deny patients their individual metaphoric interpretation of their illness is to give exclusive rights and power to the biomedical view (Scheper-Hughes, 1986; Kirmayer, 1992; Olesen, 1992; Erskine and Judd, 1994)

Nurses' Communication Skills, Feelings and 'Face-work'

Analysis of the interview data raised issues of the consequences of patients' emotional disclosure for the nurses caring for them.

Most of the nurses in the study demonstrated examples of responsive communication skills which involved the 'risk' of sustaining and escalating the emotional disclosure. These were not, however, used consistently. Previous studies have highlighted nurses' difficulties when communicating with cancer patients but have not described such responsiveness. In 1985 Maguire speculated that nurses do not possess these skills (Maguire, 1985). More recently his research suggests that it is not enough to give nurses the skill of facilitating patient disclosure (Maguire et al, 1991).

Given the amount of discussion concerning cancer nurses' emotional care of patients (Davitz and Davitz, 1980; Knight and Field, 1981; Larson, 1984), it is significant to find that the nurse participants felt anxious and underconfident in their ability to meet these needs. This is consistent with the work of Dunkel-Schetter and Wortman (1982).

The study also raised issues of the nurses' own confidence in their identity and their image of themselves as responsive and able to deal with their own feelings as well as those of their patients. This was evidenced in the pervasive 'face-work' nurses engaged in during the interview, in nurses' anxiety and worry about participating in the study and in the relationship between 'face-work' and responsive communication skills used by the nurse subjects. Some nurses were unwilling to join in the study and others withdrew after consenting to participate. Exposure of their practice on tape was a reason given for withdrawal. These findings were consistent with previous work (Craytor, 1977; Vachon, 1978; Corner, 1990). In Smith's work on the 'emotional labour' of nursing, nurses' management of their own feelings is discussed. Smith suggests that nurses suppress their feelings for their own safety (Smith, 1991). These findings do raise some interesting questions about the nature of nurses' 'face-work' and defensiveness.

It is suggested that 'face-work' is one way currently open to nurses to protect themselves from the dilemma described by Menzies Lyth in 1960 that 'by the very nature of her profession the nurse is at considerable risk of being flooded by intense and unmanageable anxiety. It is only half the story to think that this 'unmanageable anxiety' is the sheer quantity as well as the force of the feelings communicated to nurses. The whole story concerns the inner world of the nurse as well as the patient and relates to earlier life experience and infancy (Menzies Lyth, 1960). For Menzies Lyth considers that nurses are confronted by opposing sets of feelings in their work. These opposing feelings are pity, compassion and love versus hatred and resentment of the patients who arouse these strong feelings. These reflect the most basic motivations which everyone has relating to childhood experiences and strong feelings towards siblings and parents. Because of the anxiety and guilt associated with them, the feelings are pushed from consciousness and are held in check by various mechanisms of defence which serve to disguise their conscious presentation.

The stress that a nurse feels, her argument continues, is influenced by this inner world and elements remaining from infancy. Unconsciously the nurse will respond in part according to her own psychic underworld. Similarly, cancer patients and their families have an inner world which is also characterised by fantasies reminiscent of early experiences as a child – experiences with which the adult is not usually in touch, but which surface at a time of crisis and need. The overt distress and the more subtle covert messages from patients and relatives therefore increase the nurse's stress, possibly at an unconscious level.

Is it any wonder therefore, that oncology nurses who may be skilled communicators might block their own skills and use them inconsistently? The projection of strong feelings from the patient would be too much for any human unless they were themselves 'held' in a supporting, containing team (Barbanell, 1986; Wright, 1991).

In her seminal paper, *The Functioning of Social Systems as a Defence Against Anxiety*, Menzies Lyth describes the way in which the hospital situation protects the nurse from 'unmanageable anxiety'. Task-centred care with its expectation of professional and emotional detachment is one example.

It is argued that this social defence system may not necessarily exist today to provide the cover from anxiety, uncertainty and guilt that it has succeeded in providing hitherto. This would be for many reasons, including changes in planning and delivery of nursing care, cancer patients' and nurses' perceptions of emotional need and the high value and expectation cancer nurses hold concerning the provision of emotional care and support to patients.

'Face-work' is in turn a marker of the emotional cost, anxiety and personal conflicts that can ensue when nurses are caring for cancer patients. If this new 'face-work defence system' turns out sufficiently to match the individual psychic defences of the nurse outlined by Menzies Lyth, both will continue to support and feed the other.

This will not facilitate the growth, fulfilment or maturation of cancer nurses. Yet such understanding and maturity is necessary if nurses are to respond to patients' emotional needs.

Conclusions

Practical lessons are hard to draw from such a study. Consistent with the approach and theme of the work is the rejection of any one-sided attempt in the form of prescriptions for 'good communication' or 'communication skills training', to make us experts in emotional as well as clinical realities. With this in mind the following recommendations are offered.

There should be acknowledgement of the conscious and unconscious processes and consequences to nurses of dealing with the emotional needs of cancer patients. This requires commitment in principle and in practical terms if nurses are to be sustained in their care of cancer patients.

Communication skills training does have an important place, and imaginative experiential methods of teaching communication skills require development and the support of health authorities.

Nurses have a responsibility to listen and use language so that unclear, unhelpful patterns of communication no longer persist and patients can, if they wish, directly confront their negative feelings and fears at surface and deep levels and their individual voice be heard at both.

In this way cancer nurses will truly embody what Benner termed the 'helping role'.

Transcription Notation

The form of notation used throughout this study was developed by Gail Jefferson (1984). It is used in simplified form.

1. Extended square brackets mark overlap between utterances e.g.:

    N: I would ⌈like to
    P: ⌊Well I can

2. An equals sign at the end of a speaker's utterance and at the start of the next utterance indicates the absence of a discernable gap e.g.:

> N: Anyway I'll ask Doctor =
> P: = No it's alright

3. Numbers in brackets indicate pauses timed to the nearest tenth of a second. A full stop in brackets indicates a pause which is noticeable but too short to measure e.g.:

> N: I have (2.1) I need to (.) change this

4. One or more colons indicates an extension of the preceding vowel sound e.g.:

> P: Fi::ne I see::

5. Underlining indicates that words are uttered with added emphasis; words in capitals are uttered louder than the surrounding talk e.g.:

> N: I didn't say that AT ALL

6. A full stop before a word or sound indicates an audible intake of breath e.g.:

> P: It hurts . more than I thought

7. Square brackets indicate that some transcript has been deliberately omitted. Material in round brackets is clarificatory information e.g.::

> P: I told her (the patient's mother) that [ ] it's alright

8. Lines are numbered chronologically from the beginning of each complete transcript.

9. Comments non-verbal, paralinguistic, prosodic, contextual and interpretive information are given in single brackets e.g.: (quietly) (laughing) (sighing)

10. As talk does not take the form of sentences but turns, full stops are not used nor other types of conventional punctuation: commas, colons, etc.

11. Quasilexical forms are used to describe hesitation and noises e.g.: um mm er ah oh

References

Bacon P (1988) *An Exploratory Study of the Communication between Nurses and Breast Surgery Patients.* BSc dissertation, University of London.
Barbanell L H (1986) The selfless caretaker. *Psychotherapy Patient* 2(2):105–9.
Benner P (1984) *From Novice to Expert. Excellence and Power in Clinical Nursing Practice.* California: Addison-Wesley.

Blum L H (1985) Beyond medicine: Healing power in the doctor–patient relationship. *Psychological Reports* 57:399–427.

Bond S (1978) *Processes of Communication about Cancer in a Radiotherapy Department.* PhD thesis, University of Edinburgh.

Carpenter P J and Morrow G R (1986) Clinical care of cancer patients: Close interpersonal encounters of the difficult kind. *Journal of Psychosocial Oncology* 3(4, Winter):67–73.

Cassileth B, Lusk E and Miller D (1985) Psychosocial correlates of survival in advanced malignant disease. *New England Journal of Medicine* **312**:1551–5.

Cohen T (1981) Metaphor and the Cultivation of Intimacy. In: Sacks S (ed) *On Metaphor:* Chicago: University of Chicago Press.

Corner J L (1990) *An Evaluation of a Teaching Package on Nurses' Knowledge and Attitudes to Cancer and Cancer Patients.* PhD thesis, University of London.

Coupland N and Coupland J (1988) Elderly Self-Disclosure: Interactional and Intergroup Issues. *Language and Communication* **8**(2):109–33.

Cox T and McKay C (1982) Psychosocial factors and psychophysiological mechanisms in the aetiology and development of cancers. *Social Science and Medicine* **16**:381–96.

Craytor J K (1977) *A Study of Nurses' Views and Perceptions Related to Cancer Care, Cancer Patients and Cancer Nurses.* PhD thesis, University of Rochester, New York.

Davitz A and Davitz P (1980) *Nurses' Responses to Patients' Suffering.* London: Springer.

Derlaga J and Berg J H (eds) (1987) *Self-Disclosure: Theory, Research and Therapy.* New York: Plenum.

Derogatis L, Abeloff M and Melisaratos N (1979) Psychological coping mechanism and survival time in metastatic breast cancer. *Journal of the Annals of the Medical Association* **242**:1504–8.

Doan B D and Gray R E (1992) The heroic cancer patient: A critical analysis of the relationship between illusion and mental health. *Canadian Journal of Behavioral Science* **24**(2):253–66.

Drummond-Mills W (1983) *Problems Related to the Nursing Management of the Dying Patient.* MSc dissertation, University of Glasgow.

Dunkel-Schetter C and Wortman C B (1982) The interpersonal dynamics of cancer: Problems in social relationships and their impact on the patient. In: Friedman H S and DiMatteo M R (eds) *Interpersonal Issues in Health Care.* New York: Academic Press.

Erskine A and Judd D (eds) (1994) *The Imaginative Body.* London: Whurr.

Fiore N (1979) Fighting cancer – One patient's perspective. *New England Journal of Medicine* **300**:284–9.

Forrest D (1983) Analysis of nurses' verbal communication with patients. *Nursing Papers* **19**(3):48–57.

Gergen K J (1985) Social Constructionist Inquiry: Context and Implications. In: Gergen K J and Davis K E (eds) *The Social Construction of the Person.* New York: Springer.

Glaser B and Strauss A L (1965) *Awareness of Dying.* New York: Aldine.

Goffman E (1955) On face-work: An analysis of ritual elements in social interaction. *Psychiatry* **18**:213–31.

Goffman E (1959) *The Presentation of Self in Everyday Life.* Harmondsworth: Penguin.

Greer S (1983) Cancer and the Mind. *British Journal of Psychiatry* **143**:535–43.

Greer S, Morris T and Pettingale K W (1979) Psychological responses to breast cancer: Effect on outcome. *Lancet,* **2**(8146):785–7.

Greer S and Watson M (1987) Mental adjustment to cancer: Its measurement and prognostic importance. *Cancer Surveys* **6**(3):439–51.

Harre R (1986) *The Social Construction of Emotions.* Oxford: Basil Blackwell.

Hochschild A R (1979) Emotion work, feeling rules and social structure. *American Journal of Sociology* **85**(3):551–75.

Hochschild A R (1983) *The Managed Heart: Commercialisation of Human Feeling.* Berkeley: University of California Press.

Holmes S (1988) Meaningful communication: Can it enhance the quality of life? *Holistic Medicine.* **3**:195–203.

Holmes S and Dickerson J (1987) The quality of life design and evaluation of a self-assessment instrument for use with cancer patients. *International Journal of Nursing Studies* **24**(1):15–24.

Hunt M (1989) *Dying At Home: Its Basic 'Ordinariness' Displayed in Patients', Relatives' and Nurses' Talk.* PhD thesis, University of London.

James N (1993) Divisions of Emotional Labour: Disclosure and Cancer. In Fineman S (ed) *Emotion in Organizations:* 94–117. London: Sage.

Jefferson G (1984) On 'Stepwise Transition' from Talk about a 'Trouble' to Inappropriately Next Positioned Matters. In: Atkinson J and Heritage J (eds) *Structures of Social Action: Studies in Conversation Analysis.* Cambridge: Cambridge University Press.

Jensen M A (1987) Psychological factors predicting the course of breast cancer. *Journal of Personality* **55**:317–42.

Kemper T D (1981) Social constructionist and positivist approaches to the sociology of emotions. *American Journal of Sociology* **87**(2):336–62.

Kirmayer L J (1992) The body's insistence on meaning: Metaphor as presentation and representation in illness experience. *Medical Anthropology Quarterly* **6**(4):323–46.

Knight M and Field D (1981) A silent conspiracy: coping with dying cancer patients on an acute surgical ward. *Journal of Advanced Nursing* **6**:221–9.

Kreitler S, Chaitchik S and Kreitler H (1993) Repressiveness: Cause or result of cancer? *Psycho-Oncology* **2**:43–54.

Larson P J (1984) Important nurse caring behaviours perceived by patients with cancer. *Oncology Nursing Forum* **11**(6):46–50.

LeShan L and Worthington R E (1956) Personality as a factor in the pathogenesis of cancer: A review. *British Journal of Medical Psychology* **29**:49–56.

Ley P (1988) *Communicating with Patients.* London: Croom Helm.

Lichter I (1987) *Communication in Cancer Care.* London: Churchill Livingstone.

Lonnqvist J (1981) Adaptation to cancer. *Psychiatry Fennica,* Supplement, 179–88.

Maguire P (1985) The psychological impact of cancer. *British Journal of Hospital Medicine* **34**(2):100–3.

Maguire P, Booth K, Faulkner A and Elliot C (1991) *Improving Patient Disclosure of Psychological Problems.* Presented at The British Psychosocial Oncology Group Conference, London.

May C (1992) Individual care? Power and subjectivity in therapeutic relationships. *Sociology* **26**(4):589–602.

McIntosh J (1974) Processes of communication, information seeking and control associated with cancer: A selective review of the literature. *Social Science and Medicine* **8**:167–87.

McMahon R and Pearson A (1991) *Nursing as Therapy.* London: Chapman and Hall.

Menzies Lyth I (1960) A case study of the functioning of social systems as a defence against anxiety. *Human Relations* **13**(2):95–123.

Mitchell G W and Glicksman A S (1977) Cancer patients' knowledge and attitudes to cancer. *Cancer* **40**(1):61–6.

Morrow G R, Craytor J K, Brown J and Fass M (1976) Nurses' perceptions of themselves, cancer nurses, typical, ideal and cancer patients. *Perceptual and Motor Skills* **43**:1083–91.

Olesen V L (1992) Extraordinary Events and Mundane Ailments: The Contextual Dialectics of the Embodied Self. In: Ellis C and Flaherty M G (eds) *Investigating Subjectivity: Research on the Lived Experience:* pp.205–20. London: Sage.

Perakyla A (1991) Hope work in the care of seriously ill patients. *Qualitative Health Research* **1**(4),407–33.

Pettingale K W, Morris T, Greer S and Haybittle J L (1985) Mental attitudes to cancer: An additional prognostic factor. *Lancet* **1**:750.

Pistrang N and Barker C (1992) Disclosure of concerns in breast cancer. *Psycho-Oncology* **1**:183–92.

Potter J and Wetherell M (1987) *Discourse and Social Psychology: Beyond Attitudes and Behaviour.* London: Sage.

Quint J C (1965) Institutional practices of informational control. *Psychiatry*, **28**:119–32.

Rosaldo M (1984) Toward an Anthropology of Self and Feeling. In: Shweder R A and LeVine R A (eds) *Culture Theory: Essays on Mind, Self and Emotion:* 137–57. Cambridge: Cambridge University Press.

Scheper-Hughes N (1986) Speaking 'truth' to illness: Metaphors, reification and a pedagogy for patients. *Medical Anthropology Quarterly* **17**(5):137–40.

Schonfield J (1975) Psychological and life experience differences between Israeli women with benign and cancerous lesions. *Journal of Psychosomatic Research* **19**:229–34.

Shotter J and Gergen K J (eds) (1992) *Texts of Identity.* London: Sage.

Smith P (1991) The nursing process: Raising the profile of emotional care in nurse training. *Journal of Advanced Nursing* **16**:74–81.

Sontag S (1978) *Illness as a Metaphor.* Harmondsworth: Penguin.

Tait A (1986) The mastectomy experience: Two interviews examined. In: Stanley L and Scott S (eds) *Studies in Sexual Politics.* Manchester: University of Manchester.

Taylor P, Abrahams D and Hewetson M (1988) Cancer stress and personality: A correlational investigation of life events, repression sensitization and locus of control. *British Journal of Medical Psychology* **61**:179–83.

Temshok L (1985) Biopsychosocial studies on cutaneous malignant melanoma: Psychosocial factors associated with prognostic indicators, progression psychophysiology and tumour host response. *Social Science and Medicine* **20**:833–40.

Todarello O, La Pesa M W, Zaka S, Martino V and Lattanzio E (1989) Alexithymia and breast cancer. *Psychotherapy and Psychosomatics* **51**:51–5.

Uys L R (1980) Towards the development of an operational definition of the concept 'Therapeutic Use of Self'. *International Journal of Nursing Studies* **17**:175–80.

Vachon M L (1978) Motivation and stress experienced by staff working with the terminally ill. *Death Education* **2**:113–22.

Del Vecchio Good M J, Good B J, Schaffer C and Lind S E (1990) American oncology and the discourse on hope. *Culture, Medicine and Psychiatry* **14**:59–79.

Weisman A and Worden J (1975) Psychological analysis of cancer deaths. *Omega: Journal of Death and Dying* **6**:61–75.

Weisman A and Worden J W (1977) *Coping and Vulnerability.* Research Report. Boston, Massachusetts: Massachusetts General Hospital.

Wilkinson S (1991) Factors which influence how nurses communicate with cancer patients. *Journal of Advanced Nursing* **16**:677–88.

Wright H (1991) The patient, the nurse, his life and her mother: Psychodynamic influences in nurse education and practice. *Psychoanalytic Psychotherapy* **5**(2):139–49.

Chapter 11
A Comparative Study of Psychological Morbidity in Women with Screen Detected and Symptomatic Breast Cancer

Alison Farmer, Sheila Payne and Gavin Royle

Introduction

England and Wales have the highest mortality rate from breast cancer in the world with approximately 16 000 women dying from the disease each year (Cancer Research Campaign, 1991). The management of breast cancer has been the subject of debate and research for centuries, with great swings in treatment preference ranging from potions and poultices to radical surgery (De Moulin, 1989). Despite the plethora of treatments there has been little impact on mortality and even today there appears to be no consensus of opinion as far as the optimum treatment is concerned (Morris *et al*, 1992).

The psychological consequences of breast cancer have also been given a considerable amount of attention both anecdotally and empirically. The significance of the breast as an object of sexual desire and symbol of femininity, comfort and nurturing, makes the breast far more than merely a milk-producing gland on the chest wall. Anxiety, depression, sexual dysfunction, low self-esteem and poor quality of life following both diagnosis and treatment have been reported in a number of studies over the years (Bard and Sutherland, 1955; Morris *et al*, 1977, Maguire *et al*, 1978).

This early research highlighted the difficulties experienced by women with breast cancer and was responsible for some of the changes that have taken place in its management. Diagnosis and treatment are now mostly a two-stage procedure and few women have to face the horror of going to the operating theatre not knowing whether or not they will return having lost all or part of a breast. Women are more likely to be offered a choice of treatment and reconstructive surgery and to have access to a breast care nurse or cancer counsellor (Morris *et al*, 1992). The most significant change in the breast cancer field, however, must be the introduction of the National Breast Screening Programme. Breast screening, introduced in 1988 following the recommendations of the Forrest report (DHSS, 1986), offers all women aged between 50 and 64 three-yearly mammography. The aim of breast screening is to detect early invasive or non-invasive cancers that are confined to the breast tissue, as the success of treatment depends on the stage at which the cancer is detected. A woman with early breast cancer with no nodal involvement has an 87 per cent chance of surviving five years compared to a 47 per cent chance once the cancer has spread to the lymph nodes (Strax, 1984).

The early mass population studies of breast screening reported as much as a 30 per cent reduction in mortality in the screened group (Shapiro *et al*, 1982; Tabar *et al*, 1989). However, breast screening has not been without its critics. Criticism has mainly been directed at the incidence of false positive and false negative results, the unnecessary surgery and the financial cost of the programme (Gravelle *et al*, 1982; Skrabenek, 1985; Roberts, 1989). It has also been suggested that four biases – lead time, length, self-selection and over-diagnosis – may be responsible for the survival differences between women with screened and clinically-detected breast cancer (Habbema *et al*, 1983; Skrabenek, 1985).

Concern has also been expressed regarding the potential negative psychological sequelae that may arise following exposure to breast screening, including 'cancerophobia' and excessive breast self-examination (BSE) (Maguire, 1983; Roebuck, 1986). Dean *et al* (1986) interviewed women with 'normal' mammograms six months after they had attended screening and compared them to a matched random community sample. There were no significant differences between the groups, although almost 50 per cent of the screened women reported examining their breasts more than once a month. Excessive BSE following breast screening has also been reported by Bull and Campbell (1991). Ellman *et al* (1989) found significantly higher levels of anxiety in women who had false positive results and women with symptomatic benign disease compared to those routinely screened. However, at three months, only the symptomatic benign group remained significantly anxious.

The number of screen-detected cancers in this study was too small to draw any conclusions, although the authors suspected that asymptomatic screened women would find the diagnosis of breast cancer more distressing than women whose suspicions had been aroused by symptoms. Gram *et al* (1990), also studying women with false positive results, found that after 18 months the experience was regarded as a minor stress. There was, however, a degree of physical morbidity including pain and reduced sexual sensitivity in women who had excision biopsies.

Studies that have addressed the psychological aspects of breast screening have mostly excluded women who were diagnosed with cancer. Although, clinically, women with screen-detected breast cancer appeared to be more distressed than women with symptomatic breast cancer, there were few data to support this hypothesis. The lack of such data and the clinical impression was the major impetus for this study which sought to investigate whether women with screen-detected breast cancer suffered from more psychological morbidity than women with symptomatic breast cancer.

Methods

A consecutive sample of women with screen-detected breast cancer ($n=36$), and symptomatic breast cancer ($n=32$) was recruited from the breast clinics of a hospital in the Wessex Region. A group of women undergoing general surgical procedures was also included ($n=31$), to control for the effects of admission to hospital for a surgical procedure. Women with advanced cancer, previous history of malignancy or psychiatric illness were excluded from the study. The characteristics of the participants are reported in table 11.1.

Recruitment

The participants with breast cancer were approached by the investigator at the time of diagnosis, after they had been seen by the surgeon and the breast care nurse. The purpose and design of the study was explained and an appointment was made to visit the women in their own homes one week later, prior to their definitive surgery. Patients have been shown to 'put on a brave face' in the hospital situation and underestimate their true feelings, (Baum *et al*, 1990) which was the rationale behind interviewing the participants at home.

Data were collected at one week, three and six months post-diagnosis and, in the case of the control group, one day pre-operation and then three and six months later. At each interview participants completed the Hospital Anxiety and Depression scale (HADS) (Zigmond and Snaith, 1983), the Rotterdam Symptom Checklist (RSCL) (De Haes *et al*, 1983) and a Self-Esteem Linear Analogue Scale (SES) (Greer and Burgess, 1987). The participants with breast cancer also took part in a tape-recorded semi-structured interview at one week and six months post-diagnosis.

Standardised measures

Hospital Anxiety and Depression Scale

The HADS is a self-assessment tool which was specifically designed for use in non-psychiatric hospital departments. It is a 14-item scale divided into two subscales of anxiety and depression and identifies 'cases' (scores of 11–21), 'borderline' (scores of 8–10) and 'non-cases' (scores of 0–7) of clinical anxiety and depression. It was designed to exclude somatic items of anxiety and depression, which makes it particularly useful in studies with patients who have cancer. Item 8, 'I feel slowed down', could be confounded with the disease process but it is not anticipated that this would have influenced the results of this study as the participants had early breast cancer.

Table 11.1 Characteristics of study participants (Percentages in parentheses)

	Screened	Symptomatic	Control	P-value
Age				
Mean (SD)	59 (4.6)	60 (6.1)	59 (5.0)	P = 0.44
Range	50–65	50–69	51–69	
Marital status				
Married	26 (72)	24 (75)	22 (71)	P = 0.93
Single	2 (6)		1 (3)	
Widowed	4 (11)	5 (16)	4 (13)	
Divorced	4 (11)	3 (9)	4 (13)	
*Social class**				
I and II	15 (42)	16 (50)	11 (35)	P = 0.71
III, IV and V	11 (30)	10 (31)	11 (35)	
Type of cancer				
Invasive	31 (86)	27 (84)		P = 1.00
Non-invasive	5 (14)	5 (16)		
Nodal status†				
Node positive	28 (80)	21 (68)		P = 0.27
Node negative	7 (20)	10 (32)		
Breast surgery				
Mastectomy	4 (11)	16 (50)		P = 0.0005
Wide excision	32 (89)	16 (50)		
Adjuvant therapy				
DXT	20 (55)	10 (31)		P = 0.13
Chemo & DXT	0	2 (6)		
General surgery				
Varicose veins			23 (74)	
Hernia			3 (10)	
Cholecystectomy			4 (13)	
Haemorrhoidectomy			1 (3)	

* 10 screened, 6 symptomatic and 9 controls were unclassifiable
† 1 screened and 1 symptomatic patient node status unknown

Table 11.2 Sample size at each interview

	Int. 1		Int. 2		Int. 3	
Group	n	%	n	%	n	%
Screened	36	100	34	94	33	91
Symptomatic	32	100	32	100	31	96
Control	31	100	27	87	24	77

Rotterdam Symptom Checklist

The RSCL is a self-assessment 'Quality of Life' measure with two subscales of physical and psychological complaints. It was designed for use with patients who have cancer. The current version contains 18 physical and eight psychological items (Watson *et al*, 1992). It has been recommended that the HADS and the RSCL be used in conjunction with each other to improve sensitivity (Hopwood *et al*, 1991).

Self-Esteem Linear Analogue Scale

The SES consists of 15 items in the form of linear analogue scales. This tool was also specifically designed for use with patients who have cancer and is quick and easy to complete.

One of the drawbacks of standardised measures is their inability to provide rich explanatory data. Although information concerning the psychological and functional well-being of patients is obtained, they fail to take into account complex social, cognitive and environmental factors. The respondent is confined to the categories imposed by the researcher and for this reason standardised measures are best used in conjunction with an interview.

Semi-Structured Interview Schedules

The interview schedules were included to gain further information regarding pre- and postoperative adjustment and consisted of both open and closed questions. The preoperative schedule included questions regarding the participants' knowledge of breast screening, BSE habits, awareness of treatments and satisfaction with care. The postoperative interview schedule was mainly concerned with return to work/ social activities, satisfaction with information and attributions. The results of the semi-structured interview will not be reported in full, but some quotations will be used to illustrate the discussion.

Results

The results of the HADS, RSCL and SES will be reported. Data were analysed using the *Statistical Package for the Social Sciences* (SPSS). Sample size and attrition rate are presented in table 11.2.

Interview 1

Rotterdam Symptom Checklist

Psychological subscale

There were significantly more psychological complaints in the symptomatic group at the time of the first interview, Kruskal Wallace 1-way ANOVA, $P=0.001$.

Further analysis, using Mann Whitney U Test, revealed that the symptomatic group were significantly more psychologically distressed than the screened, $P=0.005$, and control groups, $P=0.0006$. (see table 11.3.)

Table 11.3 RSCL psychological subscale – Interview I

Group	n	median	U	Prob
Screened	36	6.0	353	0.005
Symptomatic	32	9.5		
Screened	36	6.0	503	0.631
Control	31	6.0		
Symptomatic	32	9.5	236	0.0006
Control	31	6.0		

Physical subscale

There were significantly more physical complaints in the symptomatic group at the time of the first interview, Kruskal Wallace 1-way ANOVA, $P=.03$.

When one group was compared against another, Mann Whitney U Test, the symptomatic group reported significantly more physical complaints than the screened group, $P=0.01$. The difference between the symptomatic and control group was not statistically significant (see table 11.4).

Table 11.4 RSCL physical subscale – Interview I

Group	n	median	U	Prob
Screened	36	6.5	371	0.011
Symptomatic	32	11.5		
Screened	36	6.5	452	0.183
Control	31	7.0		
Symptomatic	32	11.5	405	0.212
Control	31	7.0		

Self esteem linear analogue scale

The symptomatic group had lower median scores (indicating lower self esteem), at the time of the first interview. The difference, however, was not statistically significant. Kruskal Wallace 1-way ANOVA, P=0.26. There were also no statistically significant differences when one group was compared with another.

Interview 2

Rotterdam Symptom Checklist
Psychological subscale
At the time of the second interview the median scores of the symptomatic group were higher than the screened and the control groups. The difference however was not statistically significant, Kruskal Wallace 1-way ANOVA, P=0.54.

Physical subscale
Although the median scores of the control group were lower than the screened and the syptomatic groups the difference was not statistically significant, Kruskal Wallace 1-way ANOVA, P=0.80.

Self esteem linear analogue scale
There were also no statistically significant differences in self esteem between the groups, Kruskal Wallace 1 Way ANOVA, P=0.4

Interview 3

Rotterdam Symptom Checklist
Phychological subscale
At the time of the third interview the control group had slightly higher median scores on the psychological subscale than the screened and the symptomatic groups, but the difference was again not statistically significant, Kruskal Wallace 1-way ANOVA, P=0.98.

Physical subscale
The control group reported more physical complaints than the screened and the symptomatic group, however, the difference was not statistically significant, Kruskal Wallace 1-way ANOVA, P=0.28.

Self esteem linear analogue scale
Kruskal Wallace 1-way ANOVA failed to show any statistically significant differences between the groups, P=0.09.

Further analysis, comparing one group against another, showed the control group had significantly higher self esteem than the screened group, Mann Whitney U Test, P=0.03.

Hospital anxiety and depression scale

Figure 11.1 illustrates the number of cases of clinical anxiety pre and post operatively, borderline and non-cases were combined in the analysis. There were significantly more cases of clinical anxiety amongst the symptomatic group at the time of the first interview, Chi Square=6.47, P<0.03. At interview, 3 months post diagnosis, and interview 3, 6 months post diagnosis, there were no statistically significant differences between the groups.

Figure 11.2 illustrates the number of cases of clinical depression pre and post operatively, borderline and cases were combined in the analysis. There were significantly more cases of clinical depression amongst the symptomatic group at the time of the first interview, Fisher's Exact Test, P=0.01. At interview 2 and 3 there were no statistically significant differences between the groups.

Summary of results

a) At the time of the first interview, 1 week after diagnosis, the symptomatic group consistently reported more anxiety, depression, psychological and physical compaints than the screened and the control groups. The symptomatic group also reported lower self esteem, however, this failed to reach statistical significance.

b) At the time of the second interview, 3 months after diagnosis there were no statistically significant differences between the groups.

c) At the time of the 3rd interview, 6 months after diagnosis, the incidence of anxiety, depression. physical and psychological complaints was low and all three groups reported an increase in their self esteem.

Discussion

Despite both groups having early breast cancer, awaiting definitive surgery and being under the care of the same medical team, the symptomatic group reported significantly more psychological and physical morbidity than the screened. To imagine that breast screening is completely stress-free would be naïve and would contradict other studies (Bull and Campbell, 1991; Lerman *et al*, 1991). The participants were interviewed after diagnosis as it is recognised that the period between the discovery of a breast lump and diagnosis of cancer is extremely distressing (Fallowfield, 1991). For many of the symptomatic women it was the worst part of the experience:

(Symptomatic) 'Oh that is the most stressful of all, I felt awful, that is the most

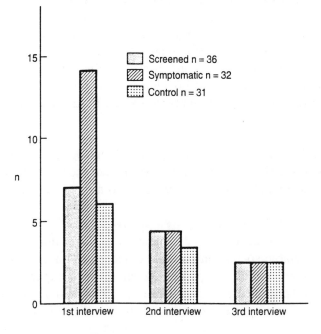

Figure 11.1   HADS Anxiety Scale

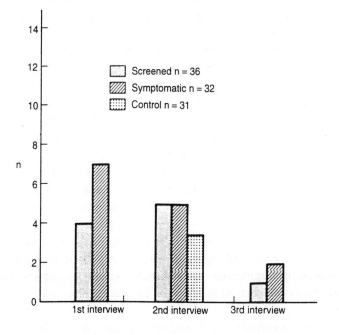

Figure 11.2   HADS Depression Scale

stressful I must say it's agonising I would rather someone came in and shot me. That fear, that is the worst part of the whole thing waiting for the results.

It was anticipated that anxiety amongst the symptomatic women would be particularly high whilst they waited for their results and it would be unfair to compare them to an asymptomatic group. However, the screened women were experiencing a similar period of uncertainty after receiving the letter recalling them to the screening assessment centre. Comparisons can be made between the two experiences:

(screened) 'well that was the worst thing that ever happened to me everything just shattered, I didn't sleep, I didn't eat, it was one of the most dreadful things we all were just shattered it was like facing up to a death sentence it was an awful thing.'

The prospect of having cancer, which threatens one's health, role and body image caused considerable social and physical dysfunction for both the screened and symptomatic women, but the psychological distress experienced by the symptomatic women continued after the 'bad news consultation' had confirmed cancer. Despite being seen by the same team of doctors, there were differences in the way the bad news was delivered. The screened women were given their diagnosis in an attractive new screening unit. The atmosphere was calm, waiting time was kept to a minimum, refreshments were available and the breast care nurse saw each patient immediately after the diagnosis was given by the doctor. The symptomatic women were seen in a busy breast clinic, for new and follow-up patients, in a radiotherapy department. Although an attempt was made to see women waiting for results quickly, there were often inevitable delays. It was hoped that, by interviewing the women one week later and in their own homes, the adverse effects of the clinic experience would be reduced.

Apart from the difference in environment there was also a difference in the way the bad news was delivered. When the screened women were given the diagnosis, the emphasis was placed by the doctor on the early stage of the cancer. During the research interviews the screened women mentioned how small the cancer was, the advantages of early detection and the benefits of breast screening. As far as they were concerned, the cancer had been found, treated and would be no further trouble:

(screened) 'The doctor did say that once I went back again that she really thinks that once that is removed then hopefully I will never see them again, I am very lucky that it has been caught early. At first they mention cancer and then when it is explained to you how small it is and how early it is then you can see clearer.'

Cancer was no longer a serious life-threatening disease, its significance had been minimised. There had been a process of cognitive adaptation. The experience had become a positive one, perhaps to avoid cognitive dissonance. The following comment, made by the same participant who said that the letter of recall was 'the worst thing that ever happened to me', illustrates this point:

(screened) 'Oh yes definitely, oh I think it [screening] was absolutely 100 per cent oh yes because, um, you don't really want to be finding lumps you want to go and have them out before then and it has taken the terror out of it for me. This is one of the things that you might find very odd but I was much more frightened about breast cancer before I had this than I am now.'

The symptomatic women were more likely to mention recurrence of their disease and were worried that the doctor had not been more reassuring. They were not concerned with what the doctor said, but what he or she did not say:

(symptomatic) 'The only thing is, I have since thought this is early breast cancer but he didn't give me any reassurance at all he didn't say we have caught it early and what the chances are, he didn't reassure me in any way and tell me what the chances are of a full recovery, I would have liked him to have spoken about that side of things. I did think that if it had been caught early that he might have been a bit more reassuring.'

There is evidence to suggest that the style of the bad news consultation, the attitude of the surgeon and the language used play a crucial part in patient adjustment (Fallowfield et al, 1990; Shapiro et al, 1992). Shapiro et al found that women who were given results of mammography from a non-worried physician recalled more information, reported lower levels of state anxiety and felt that their situation was far less severe than did those that were given results by a worried physician.

A further explanation for the psychological distress amongst the symptomatic women may have been that, as a group, more had mastectomies than the screened women (see table 11.1). There has been a long-standing assumption that the cause of psychological morbidity in women with breast cancer was the mastectomy (Renneker and Cutler, 1952); however, there is now evidence to suggest that this assumption is incorrect. In a study by Fallowfield et al (1986) there was no difference in psychological morbidity between women who had mastectomies and those who had lumpectomies.

The main concern of the women in this study was to go on living, not the extent of their surgery:

(symptomatic) 'All I can think of is saving my life, I just won't look at it.'

(screened) 'No, if it had to be that would be it, I wouldn't mind if it had to be, you know, I wouldn't mind. The thing is for it to go and you to go on living and be healthy, that is the main thing.'

One of the potential benefits of breast screening is the reduction in the number of mastectomies that will need to be performed. This may have led to the surgeon assuming that screened women would not want to even consider mastectomy. Not only were the screened women less likely to have mastectomies but they were less likely to have been offered the choice. Failure to discuss mastectomy with the screened women further minimises the significance of the disease. The message they received was that a minor problem requires only minor surgery. However, there were some screened women for whom mastectomy would have been the preferred option:

> (screened) 'I would much rather have that done [mastectomy] and finished with if that was necessary but it wasn't, well we both agreed that he knows what he is doing . . . I felt that maybe he was trying to protect me in some way.'

> (screened) 'Sometimes I think that doctors don't really believe you when you say I'm not bothered by how much you take just so long as you take it all, and I wonder whether the doctors believe you because so many women are worried about losing their breasts, but me, I'd rather lose the cancer. This is why I was sorry when he did the biopsy that he didn't take a bigger area and then do it all in one go, not if it is going to make quite sure that it is gone once and for all, because I don't want to have surgery and then take tablets and have radiotherapy. I did try to make this plain.'

Involving patients in decisions and offering them a choice of treatment has been shown to reduce psychological morbidity (Morris and Royle, 1988). It should not be assumed that the screened women differ in their desire to be involved and it is clear from the interviews that they did not always receive the treatment they wanted.

Both the screened and the symptomatic women attempted to find out further information regarding their diagnosis and treatment. The main source of information was the media. Media coverage of breast screening tends to be extremely positive. It emphasises the benefits of early detection. This, in turn, has an adverse effect on the symptomatic women as it emphasises the negative side of waiting until a breast lump appears. The positive media coverage of screening acts as a further source of reassurance and minimisation. Family and friends also read the media coverage of breast screening and may have been present when the diagnosis was given. They may also minimise the significance of the disease:

> (screened) 'If I can just quote my husband who had a very bad cough in the summer, he said to me, "Well, you know you are not paying proper attention to my cough, when you had that tiny bit of cancer we were all supposed to be being sympathetic and it was nothing as bad as what I have got at the moment," and I think that has tended to be my family's attitude, which I think actually is quite a healthy one.'

Although the symptomatic women reported considerable psychological morbidity at the first interviews, in the later interviews, at three and six months, psychological morbidity was low in all groups.

The sample size in this study was small and the results should be treated with caution. Recruitment took place in a specialist breast unit with a breast care nurse and a specific ward that admitted all the patients with breast cancer and was staffed by nurses who were able to talk to the patients about their worries. Patients were also given excellent written information. It is clear that not all clinics or hospitals will have such facilities and patients elsewhere may not adjust as well. It should also be pointed out that women who attend breast screening are a self-selecting group. They tend to be of higher social class and therefore less likely to suffer from psychiatric illness. It is not anticipated that this affected the results of this study as there was no significant difference in social class between the groups.

Conclusion

Fears that women with screen-detected breast cancer would experience more psychological morbidity than women with symptomatic breast cancer appear to be unfounded. Screened women appear not to see breast cancer as a life-threatening condition, but as something that can be caught early and cured. They are reassured by the terminology used in the 'bad news consultation', the surgeon's affect, media coverage and the attitude of significant others. All these factors lead to minimisation of their disease. It is possible that psychological morbidity was low because they may have felt obliged to be grateful to screening and for having their breast cancer detected early, that gratitude making it difficult to volunteer the true extent of their distress, even in a confidential research setting. Because psychological distress was not volunteered it does not mean that it does not exist (Fallowfield et al, 1987).

The introduction of breast screening has given health professionals the chance to be optimistic with a group of patients who were previously seen as having little hope. It is more comfortable for the health professional to minimise the significance of the disease and imply that it will cause no further problems. It is still possible, however, to give a positive message without giving false reassurance.

Minimisation is a useful coping strategy as long as women remain disease-free (Payne, 1990). Although there is little doubt that breast screening will have some impact on mortality, there will be some women who go on to develop a recurrence and eventually die. Women who were convinced that their cancer would not return may feel angry and let down by a service that they believed promised them a cure. They may ignore signs of recurrence and we may see breast-screening attendance falling as women lose faith in the service.

Women need more information about the nature of breast cancer, why they have been invited, how participation will affect them, the incidence and meaning of positive and negative results and what action will be taken (Marteau, 1990). It is essential that women realise that they must continue to be breast-aware and seek help immediately there is any sign of recurrence. It is desirable that women are offered a choice of treatment whenever this is feasible. Finally, as it is likely that a considerable number of screen-detected breast cancer patients will subsequently experience a recurrence, an important area for future research would be their transitions in understanding of the disease and its psychological impact.

Acknowledgements

I would like to thank, very much, all the women who agreed to take part in this study. I would also like to thank the Wessex Cancer Trust for their generous financial support.

References

Bard M and Sutherland A M (1955) Psychological impact of cancer and its treatment: IV adaptation to radical mastectomy. *Cancer* **8**: 656–72.

Baum M, Ebbs S R, Fallowfield L J and Fraser S C A (1990) Measurement of quality of life in advanced breast cancer. *Acta Oncologica* **29**: 391–5.

Bull A R and Campbell M J (1991) Assessment of the psychological impact of a breast screening programme. *The British Journal of Radiology* **64**: 510–15.

Cancer Research Campaign (1991) *Breast Cancer Factsheets*, No 6 and No 7. London: Cancer Research.

Dean C, Roberts M M, French K and Robinson S (1986) Psychiatric morbidity after screening for breast cancer. *Journal of Epidemiology and Community Health* **40**:71–5.

DHSS (1986) *Breast Cancer Screening* (Forrest Report). London: HMSO.

Ellman R, Angeli N, Christians A, Moss S, Chamberlain J and Maguire P (1989) Psychiatric morbidity associated with screening for breast cancer. *British Journal of Cancer* **60**(5): 781–4.

Fallowfield L (1991) *Breast Cancer*. London: Routledge.

Fallowfield L J, Baum M and Maguire G P (1986) Effects of breast conservation on psychological morbidity associated with diagnosis and treatment of early breast cancer. *British Medical Journal* **293**: 1331–4.

Fallowfield L J, Baum M and Maguire G P (1987) Addressing the psychological needs of the conservatively treated breast cancer patient: A discussion paper. *Journal of the Royal Society of Medicine* **80**: 696–700.

Fallowfield L J, Hall A, Maguire G P and Baum M (1990) Psychological outcomes of different treatment policies in women with early breast cancer outside a clinical trial. *British Medical Journal* **301**: 575–80.

Gram I T, Lund E and Slenker S E (1990) Quality of life following a false positive mammogram. *British Journal of Cancer* **62**: 1018–22.

Gravelle H, Simpson P and Chamberlain J (1982) Breast cancer screening and health service costs. *Journal of Health Economics* **1**: 185–207.

Greer S and Burgess C (1987) A self-esteem measure for patients with cancer. *Psychology and Health* 1: 327–40.

Habbema J D F, Van Oortmarssen G J and Van Putten D J (1983) An analysis of survival differences between clinically and screen-detected cancer patients. *Statistics in Medicine* 2: 279–85.

De Haes J C J M, Pruyn J F A, and Knippenberg F C E (1983) Klachtenlijst voor kankerpatienten: Eerste ervaringen. *Nederlands Tijdschrift voor de Psychologie* 38:403–22.

Hopwood P, Howell A and Maguire P (1991) Screening for psychiatric morbidity in patients with advanced breast cancer: Validation of two self-report questionnaires. *British Journal of Cancer* 64: 353–6.

Lerman C, Trock B, Rimer B, Jepson C, Brody D and Boyce A (1991) Psychological side-effects of breast cancer screening. *Health Psychology* 10 (4): 259–67.

Maguire G P, Lee E G, Bevington D J, Kuchemann C S, Crabtree R J, and Cornell C E (1978) Psychiatric problems in the first year after mastectomy. *British Medical Journal* 1: 963–5.

Maguire P G (1983) Possible psychiatric complications of screening for breast cancer. *British Journal of Radiology* 56 (664): 284 (Abstract).

Marteau T (1990) Reducing the psychological costs. *British Medical Journal* 301: 26–8.

Morris T, Greer S and White P (1977) Psychological and social adjustment to mastectomy: A two-year follow-up study. *Cancer* 40: 2381–7.

Morris J and Royle G T (1988) Offering patients a choice of surgery for early breast cancer: A reduction in anxiety and depression in patients and their husbands. *Social Science and Medicine* 27(11): 1257–62.

Morris J, Farmer A and Royle G (1992) Recent changes in the surgical management of T1/2 breast cancer in England. *European Journal of Cancer* 28A(10): 1709–12.

De Moulin (1989) *A Short History of Breast Cancer.* Dordrecht: Kluwer Academic Publishers Group.

Payne S (1990) Coping with palliative chemotherapy. *Journal of Advanced Nursing* 15:652–8.

Renneker R and Cutler M (1952) Psychological problems of adjustment to cancer of the breast. *Journal of the American Medical Association* 148: 833–8.

Roberts M M (1989) Breast screening: Time for a rethink? *British Medical Journal* 299: 1153–5.

Roebuck E J (1986) Mammography and screening for breast cancer. *British Medical Journal* 292: 223–6.

Shapiro S, Venet P, Strax P and Roeser R (1982) Ten to fourteen-year effect of breast cancer screening on mortality. *Journal of The National Cancer Institute* 69: 349–55.

Shapiro D E, Boggs S R, Melamed B G and Graham-Pole J (1992) The effect of varied physician affect on recall, anxiety and perceptions in women at risk for breast cancer: An analogue study. *Health Psychology* 11 (1): 61–6.

Skrabenek P (1985) False premises and false promises of breast cancer screening. *Lancet* ii: 316–20.

Strax P (1984) Mass screening for control of breast cancer. *Cancer* 53: 665–70.

Tabar L, Fagerberg G, Duffy S W and Day N E (1989) The Swedish two county trial of mammographic screening for breast cancer. *Journal of Epidemiology and Community Health* **43**: 107–14.

Watson M, Law M, Maguire G P, Robertson B, Greer S, Bliss J M and Ibbotson T (1992) Further development of a quality of life measure for cancer patients: The Rotterdam symptom checklist (revised). *Psycho-Oncology* **1**: 35–44.

Zigmond A S and Snaith R P (1983) The hospital anxiety and depression scale. *Acta Psychiatr. Scand.* **67**. 361–70.

Section Five

Physical Problems: Consequences for Nursing Care

Chapter 12
The Palliative Management of Fungating Malignant Wounds: Preparatory Work
Patricia Grocott

Introduction

The purpose of this chapter is to present the steps taken from the identification of a clinical problem of fungating wounds to the formulation of the research questions for a research proposal. Through this process the researcher seeks to clarify the problem in her own mind, to determine that the problem justifies the research, to compare her perceptions with that of other practitioners and to ensure that previous work is utilised and built upon.

The background to the problem in terms of pathophysiology, presentation and treatment options will therefore be described, together with its incidence and clinical significance to patients and practitioners. Evidence will also be presented of a lack of substantiation of the research by others. The origins of this project are rooted in the researcher's hospice-based palliative care experience. The values and influences which have shaped the formulation of the research questions will be acknowledged so that, following the 'critical tradition' of research, the consistency of the research problem with clinical practice and the worth of the inquiry are both subjected to critical review by knowledgeable practitioners.

Background to the Problem: the Development of a Fungating Wound

Fungating malignant wounds develop when tumour cells infiltrate and erode through the skin. The term *fungating* is used to describe the development and progression of the wound which may be proliferating and/or ulcerating (Mortimer, 1993). Tumour extension is via the uninterrupted spread of malignant cells between tissue planes, along blood and lymph capillaries and perineural spaces (Willis, 1973; Mosley, 1988; Love, 1990). Fungating wounds may develop on a number of sites, the breast being the most common (Sims and Fitzgerald, 1985; Ivetic, 1991; Thomas, 1992; Mortimer, 1993). Cancers of the lung, stomach, head and neck, uterus, kidney, ovary, colon, bladder, melanoma and lymphoma also have this potential (Mortimer, 1993).

Tumour Vasculature, Hypoxia and Tissue Necrosis

Deficiencies in solid tumour vasculature and blood flow are recognised factors which affect the success of radiation and chemotherapy regimes in controlling tumour growth and consequently the potential for fungation. The hypoxic regions within a tumour are attributed to fluctuations in the blood supply and cell perfusion. These arise from abnormalities in the structure of the vessels and also their distribution. Absence of a lymphatic system for interstitial tissue drainage may compound the situation when interstitial fluid pressures exceed extravascular pressures, leading to the collapse of vessels. Under these conditions, rapid cell proliferation may result in an acidic pH of extracellular fluid which affects the tension within blood cells and can interfere with the clotting mechanism, making the blood more susceptible to coagulation. Overall, the temporary or permanent occlusion of blood vessels together with variations in the proximity of blood vessels to tissues results in a reduced potential for oxygen diffusion (Chaplin, 1992).

The mechanisms related to tumour vasculature, blood flow and tissue oxygenation are complex and have formed the focus of multidisciplinary research studies with the aim of modifying the vasculature in order to improve cancer therapy (Chaplin, 1992; Hirst, 1992). Tissue hypoxia in a fungating wound is significant because of the consequential loss of tissue viability and necrosis. Anaerobic and aerobic bacteria proliferate in these conditions, giving rise to the characteristic symptoms of malodour and profuse exudate. The latter may be attributed to bacterial enzymes (proteases) and their assistance in tissue breakdown and liquefaction (Cutting and Harding, 1994). In addition, capillary fragility may give rise to bleeding (Saunders and Regnard, 1989; Regnard and Tempest, 1992; Thomas, 1992).

Presentation and Palliative Management

Patients with fungating wounds present with locally advanced, metastatic or recurrent disease (Mosley, 1988). Diagnosis is based on histological assessment and the management aim is to control tumour growth, arrest surface haemorrhage and promote healing whenever possible (Bates, 1984; Hoskin, 1993; Mortimer, 1993). Treatment protocols may involve one or more of the following: surgery (Baum *et al*, 1993) radiotherapy (Hoskin, 1993), neutron therapy (NACNEWS, 1993; Brennan *et al*, 1994; Skolyszewski *et al*, 1994; Stannard *et al*, 1994), low power laser therapy (Humzah *et al*, 1992), hormone manipulation or chemotherapy (MacDonald, 1993a; Kearsley, 1994). The adoption of strict lines of demarcation between curative and palliative approaches is considered inappropriate, as disease-modifying treatments can be used palliatively to enhance quality of life. Treatment selection is based on balancing effects which will cause minimal harm and maximum benefit to the patient (Mosley, 1988; MacDonald, 1993b).

The literature emphasises that the presence of an extensive fungating wound does not necessarily represent an intractable problem. Clinicians promote the use of invasive palliative measures in order to avoid the unpleasant consequences of an open and deteriorating wound. Excision, for example, of an advanced fungating breast tumour followed by closure with a myocutaneous flap can give the patients several months of a near-normal life, free at any rate from the symptoms identified (Baum *et al*, 1993; Miller *et al*, 1993).

In the absence of a response to palliative measures, the tumour cells extend unchecked along the pathways cited earlier, resulting in wounds that are continually enlarging, irregular in shape, necrotic and exuding. Patients have to live with these wounds with local measures as the remaining options. These take the form of wound dressings, topical haemostatic agents, topical Metronidazole and systemic medications for the control of symptoms such as pain, bleeding or infection (Regnard and Tempest, 1992; Hoy, 1993; Miller et al, 1993; Moody and Grocott, 1993; Mortimer, 1993).

The Scale of the Problem in Terms of Incidence or Prevalence

There is an immediate difficulty in using incidence as a criterion for justifying this study. The precise incidence of fungating malignant wounds is unknown, as data are estimated rather than derived from population-based cancer registries. Ivetic, for example, addressed the issue of incidence in her sociological case study by asking doctors and nurses to recall the numbers of patients they had cared for with such wounds. Her study sample comprised a small group of nurses from each of the following: a terminal care unit, a specialist cancer hospital and a community unit. The nurses' replies varied for example from 1–3 patients per month (10 nurses), to 10–12 per month (2 nurses), through to 16 per month (1 nurse). Expressions such as 'a lot' (3 nurses), 'loads' (1 nurse), and 'many' (1 nurse) were also used. The doctors from the same units reported that patients with fungating wounds constituted a less frequent feature of their practice (Ivetic, 1991).

Respondents in Thomas' (1992) survey were asked how many fungating wounds they had seen over the previous four weeks and to indicate if the figure was typical of an average month. They were also asked to estimate how many fungating wounds they had encountered during the previous year. Of 114 respondents (out of a total of 328 questionnaires distributed) a monthly total of 295 fungating wounds had been seen and an annual total of 2417, the majority in radiotherapy and oncology units. Thomas concluded that these figures reflect a significant incidence.

Although population-based cancer registries provide detailed regional data on the incidence of and mortality rates for different cancers for health-care planning in many countries, few data exist on the prevalence of cancer symptoms (Vainio, 1991). Point-prevalence studies can be useful in establishing the extent of a problem in support of a researcher's hunch, as demonstrated by McMahon (1994). However, Thomas' data (1992) were accumulated from a number of locations; therefore, to make a case for this research project using magnitude of incidence or point-prevalence as criteria is problematic. Overall, on the incidence data alone the project could not be justified. Other factors needed to be considered.

The Clinical Significance of the Problem in Terms of Physical and Psychological Distress

Although the issue of incidence is unclear, the clinical significance of the problem in terms of physical and psychological distress is illustrated repeatedly in the literature (Sims and Fitzgerald, 1985; Bale and Harding, 1987; Thomas, 1989, 1992; Ivetic 1991). The following quotation from Finlay (1991) is a vivid description of the physical problem of a fungating wound and its impact on the patient:

> . . . the visible marker of disease that literally eats through the body surface . . . the patient will be embarrassed by the smell of necrotic tissue, by soiling and oozing from the tumour surface and by the indignity of having a sensitive part of the body destroyed . . .

Case studies by Fitzgerald (in Sims and Fitzgerald, 1985) and Woodhouse (1992), for example, describe this embarrassment vividly. Fitzgerald also conveys the consequent isolation endured through not being able to share the problems with professional carers, let alone friends. Sims and Fitzgerald's (1985) study illustrates a patient's fear in relation to a malignant wound, as well as advancing disease.

Psychological distress may also extend to the family (Ivetic, 1991; Lister, 1991; Neal, 1991, Thomas, 1992). Bennett (1985) and Preston and Griffen (1989) give some indication of the way in which the family is drawn into an ever-increasing burden of caring, including practical wound management. Doyle (1987) describes the distressing associations of smell that may linger with the family after the patient has died.

Some authors identify limitations for the performance of dressings in relation to fungating wounds because of the complexity of the wound, the size, the irregular shape or location. These observations assume particular clinical significance because of the role dressings play in these patients' care. Bennett (1985) for example described the difficulty of dressing a discharging wound located under the chin, with the dressings needing two or three changes a day either by the patient or by nurses. Preston and Griffen (1989) identified a problem in finding a comfortable and effective dressing for a patient with a bulbous tumour on the clavicle which exuded large amounts of serosanguinous fluid, was hypersensitive to pressure and close to a tracheostomy tube and ties. Neal (1991) addressed the limitations of dressings in relation to odour, pruritus and exudate control:

A stoma bag can be useful, but it has limited application: not many cancers fungate through body surfaces where it is possible to fix a bag, let alone get a good seal.

Clark (1992) described the demoralisation associated with heavily discharging wounds and proposed that semi-permeable films may secure dressings and prevent seepage. With wounds such as those depicted in the photographs that accompany her article, it is difficult to see how this application could be made. Clark was also critical of the need for daily dressings in the management of fungating wounds but did not address the dilemma that conditions at the wound site, the rate of tissue liquefaction and bacterial burden, may require a daily dressing regime (Bolton and van Rijswijk, 1991).

The problems encountered by Woodhouse (1992) in the management of a breast wound included leakage of profuse exudate and persistent malodour, both of which distressed the patient. Woodhouse was faced with the difficulty of finding an alternative to frequent changes of gamgee and incontinence pads as a means of managing the exudate.

The approach taken by the researcher to the management of a fungating nodule on the neck was to introduce an individually moulded wound support system in foam latex as an accessory to alginate and gauze dressings. The system was developed by a make-up artist when a number of attempts at fixing a dressing to the site in order to contain the exudate had failed. Family life had broken down, necessitating the patient's admission to a hospice where a disproportionate amount of nursing time was spent on re-dressing and re-padding the wound. The individually moulded system brought the problems under control and the patient resumed out-patient status until his overall condition deteriorated (Grocott, 1992a). In a single-case study of a patient with a fungating breast wound, the main problems identified by the patient included: pain and discomfort from the removal of dressings and tape, odour, uncontrolled exudate with related problems of the integrity of dressings and soiling of clothes, bleeding at dressing changes and restrictions on the patient's daily life from district nurse visits. A change in wound management, which involved the application of absorbent, semi-occlusive dressings applied with medical adhesive and removed with a solvent, improved the patient's well-being but was not a complete solution to the maintenance of an intact dressing (Grocott, 1992b).

Banks and Jones (1993) described the problem of controlling the purulent, offensive exudate from a nasal carcinoma, the situation being compounded by the absence of a wound bed, so that exudate ran into the patient's mouth; the wound was also increasing in size. They were able to control the patient's problems to an extent by using a combination of dressings. Boardman *et al* (1993) encountered difficulties with containing the exudate and smell from a metastatic lesion in the shoulder, the patient being particularly distressed by the staining of his clothes and the odour. Based on this literature, an argument in favour of the research could be made on grounds of clinical significance whereby patients with fungating wounds represent extreme cases (Yin, 1989). From the researcher's clinical practice, the significance of the problem could be assessed in terms of extreme physical and psychological distress as experienced by patients and families and limited success in overcoming this distress. The problems were recurring and not con-fined to the occasional single case. The question raised therefore was not whether the topic should be researched but rather who was conducting the research and where?

The subject was expected to be included in the priorities for research by cancer and palliative care practitioners. This expectation is based on the commitment within the specialty of Palliative Care to control the symptoms in relation to advanced disease. The domain of the specialty, as defined by the World Health Organisation, is:

> the active total care of patients whose disease is not responsive to curative treatment. Control of pain, of other symptoms, and of psychological, social and spiritual problems, is paramount . . . Many aspects of palliative care are also applicable earlier in the course of the illness in conjunction with anticancer treatment (WHO, 1990)

Research in Palliative Care is therefore directed at symptom control and psychosocial issues as opposed to tumour growth and regression. It is applicable not only for the patient who is dying of their disease but also for those undergoing treatment who may experience symptoms and psychosocial needs (Clinch and Schipper, 1993; Doyle *et al*, 1993). However, the literature on symptom distress in cancer and palliative care patients includes studies which suggest that fungating wounds do not present a significant problem to patients and practitioners.

Shared Perception of Clinical Significance with Practitioners in the Field

In a prospective study of symptom control by Higginson and McCarthy (1987), fungating wounds did not feature as a main category symptom, but may have been included in an 'other' category. They may have featured, however, in a hospital survey of distressing symptoms in dying patients and their families by Hockley *et al* (1988) but are not specified as such – of 26 patients in the study two reported malodorous wounds quite separately from 16 who reported pressure sores. Similarly, there was no mention of wounds in a discussion paper on controlling symptoms in advanced cancer by Walsh and West (1988). Malignant wounds were not included as an item on a symptom distress scale (modified from the McCorkle and Young

Symptom Distress Scale) for cancer patients (McCorkle and Young, 1978; Holmes, 1991). McCorkle and Young (1978) however, indicate that their scale includes only symptoms that are likely to be of concern to the majority of patients.

The surveys that have been undertaken into priorities for education and research in cancer and palliative care in North America do not identify this topic as a key area for research. The Delphi survey on research priorities in cancer nursing by Oberst (1978) revealed an item in the first round which is directly relevant for fungating wounds entitled: 'Find more effective measures to prevent or control odor from wound or other drainage'. However, the question was eliminated in the second round with problems such as pain control, prevention and symptom control in relation to stomatitis assuming greater priority (Oberst, 1978).

Following a review of cancer nursing research by Grant and Padilla (1983), the authors made recommendations for the generation of studies to guide practice with the goal of making an impact on the morbidity, mortality and quality of life of cancer patients. They specified seven broad areas, one of which focused on 'nursing interventions to decrease the negative impact of the disease itself on patient health' and included topics such as lymphoedema and wound odours.

Oberst's (1978) Delphi study was partially replicated in Canada ten years on by Degner (1987). Following the first-round questionnaires, a topic considered important to patients and ranked ten out of fifteen referred to distressing symptoms associated with cancer and included odour:

Determine methods for preventing and treating distressing symptoms (such as fatigue, shortness of breath, edema, and odor) associated with cancer or its treatment.

The same topic was ranked fourteen out of fifteen as one of value for nurses. When the priority areas were narrowed to five, it was dropped, while stomatitis and anticipatory nausea emerged as the key research items (Degner, 1987).

In the UK, Wilson-Barnett and Raiman in *Nursing Issues and Research in Terminal Care* (1988) identified key areas for terminal care nursing and research and included a nursing function in relation to helping patients to cope with illness or potential health problems. In the same text, Thomas (1988) reviewed the nursing implications of enabling patients to cope with physically distressing symptoms other than pain. She included impaired wound healing in relation to ulcerating metastatic lesions, fistulae and pressure sores as one of nine concepts of physical symptoms for future investigation.

The survey by Copp and Dunn (1993) of common problems encountered when caring for the dying in acute, community and hospice settings found that the most frequent problems identified by the nurses across the three settings were physical, but they were not perceived as being correspondingly difficult to manage. The subcategories of physical problems included topics such as pain, weakness, nutrition and elimination. Only the hospice nurses cited 'skin problems' as a 'most difficult subcategory' to manage and it is assumed that malignant wounds were included amongst other conditions such as pressure sores.

Recent overviews of cancer and palliative care research priorities by Wilson-Barnett and Richardson (1993) in general and within the Department of Nursing Studies at King's College London did, however, name malignant wounds as a priority research area, indicating sustained interest in the topic since 1988.

A Delphi survey has been launched by the Macmillan Practice Development Unit at the Royal Marsden Hospital, London to identify ten research priorities for cancer palliative care for each of the disciplines involved in the specialty. It will be interesting to see if fungating wounds reach the final round of the nursing research priorities (*Nursing Times*, 1994).

There are a number of complex issues in relation to the interpretation of survey and review data which are beyond the scope of this chapter. Exploration of this aspect of the literature is also not exhaustive but the selected surveys in relation to cancer and palliative care indicate that as far as research priorities are concerned, fungating wounds may feature in the early round of topic identification but are dropped in the short-listing process. This may suggest that the priority topics which are likely to affect the whole population of cancer and palliative care patients are bound to take precedence over a problem that affects a small group within the population. It also suggests that the priority topics have not been fully researched (Copp and Dunn, 1993).

Apparent variations in professional interest in the topic may relate to the issue of incidence discussed earlier, whereby many nurses may not see fungating wounds. An alternative explanation may be that for some practitioners the presence of a wound is not a significant issue whereas pain, for example, is; just as for some patients, an extensive wound has little impact (Neal, 1991). In addition, where healing is not an achievable goal, the wound may assume less clinical importance for some than for others. Since 1992 there has been an increasing amount of published material on fungating wounds, including the case histories cited earlier and general articles (Banks and Jones, 1993; Boardman *et al*, 1993; Collinson, 1993; Fairburn, 1993, 1994; Fear, 1993; Grocott, 1993; Moody and Grocott, 1993; Bycroft, 1994).

A further indicator of professional interest in fungating wounds was found in the preliminary stages of this project when the researcher canvassed and gained support for the research in principle from key practitioners across the UK. Sources of names and addresses were the current *Hospitals and Health Services Yearbook* (IHSM, 1993) and the *Directory of Hospice and Palliative Care Services* (Hospice Information Service, 1994). The National Council for Hospice and Specialist Palliative Care Services also endorsed the need for the project and made their own submission to the House of Commons Select Committee on Health Priority Setting in the NHS, for an extension of the Drug Tariff to include large and absorbent dressings for patients with fungating wounds and lymphoedema (NCHSPCS, 1993).

From this it is apparent that the study has not previously been conducted.

A Lack of Substantiation by Other Researchers

Ivetic (1991) presented evidence in her study that patient care in relation to fungating wounds is not based on clinical criteria or scientific knowledge. She found that clinicians based their choices for wound management on a range of institutional, social, psychological and economic factors. She also concluded that patients' perceptions of their wounds, including wound treatments, have not been studied. Ivetic speculated that fungating wounds have not been studied because the nature and treatment of the condition are difficult areas to study and, as a result of their non-uniformity, are not amenable to observation through scientific methods.

The literature that does address wound management for fungating wounds supports her findings to some extent and reveals a conflict in approaches with a lack of substantiation of either approach.

A significant change in wound management came in the early 1960s with the development of moist wound healing theory (MWHT), the essence of which is that a moist rather than a dry wound environment promotes optimal healing (Winter, 1962). A review of the literature since the adoption of MWHT into clinical practice reveals concerted efforts by health care companies to develop the 'ideal wound dressing', as well as an increase in experiential and research knowledge on wound healing.

In comparison, the literature in relation to fungating wounds is limited (in spite of the increase in publications mentioned earlier) and presents two divergent methods of wound management. One favours 'wet to dry regimes' and includes the now controversial use of antiseptics; the other is underpinned by MWHT. The debate on the use of antiseptics centres on *in vitro* studies of their damaging effects on human fibroblasts and the consequent impairment of the wound healing process (Brennan *et al*, 1986; Deas *et al*, 1986). As has been stated already, the main concern for fungating wounds may not be regeneration but rather the removal of necrotic tissue and bacteria, together with the control of odour, exudate and bleeding. The indications are, however, that antiseptics are denatured in the presence of pus and that the debriding action of solutions such as eusol and hydrogen peroxide is minimal and may be attributed to mechanical effects which, in themselves, may be traumatic (Thomas, 1989).

The first approach, the use of wet to dry dressings and antiseptics, is recommended by Hanratty, for example, in the book entitled *Palliative Care of the Terminally Ill* (1989). He prescribes the following list of cleansing agents: Eusol, hydrogen peroxide, Chlorhexidine, Povidone Iodine and Metronidazole. The rationale for using these products, apart from the Metronidazole, is not given. Robbins (1989), a nurse lecturer in hospice care, also proposes Chlorhexidine and includes Cetrimide, yoghurt, Streptokinase/Streptodornase and normal saline. Recommendations for wound coverings include gauze or gamgee (which may be soaked in one of the solutions), foam elastomer, paraffin gauze, colostomy bags, charcoal dressings and cellophane for wounds which leak. She also advises that a patient's request for a single room is understandable.

In *Therapeutics in Terminal Cancer*, Twycross and Lack (1990) explained their management protocols for malignant ulcers, but their sources of information are not referenced. The stated goal of treatment is the control of malodour. They propose that practitioners should consider the use of hydrogen peroxide 3 per cent, Povidone Iodine, sodium hypochlorite, charcoal dressings, air fresheners, systemic antibiotics and, if all else fails, benzoyl peroxide 10-20 per cent soaks as a powerful oxidising agent covered by surgical pads and clingfilm. The authors advise that:

. . . occasionally a patient may complain of burning in the ulcer while the dressing is being changed . . .

but they are reassuring that this subsides within 30 minutes.

Lethem (1993) in her contribution to the third edition of *The Management of Terminal Malignant Disease* discusses the management of fungating wounds under the general heading of skin problems. The characteristics of the 'ideal wound dressing' are described in terms of promoting wound healing. When intractable wound management problems are encountered such as an extensive, exuding fungating wound that is infected, the use of antiseptics/bacteriostatics is recommended instead of the new generation dressing materials, mainly for cost reasons. Again, a notable feature of this chapter is the absence of references or data to support the interventions proposed.

In the 1986 edition of *A Guide to Symptom Relief in Advanced Cancer*, authors such as Regnard and Davies pointed out that many unrelated treatments have been recommended for the management of malignant ulcers and advocated simple methods. They advised practitioners to avoid the use of antiseptics and topical antibiotics and proposed that dressings should provide a moist wound environment. These recommendations are carried forward to the third edition (Regnard and Tempest, 1992).

A number of practitioners support the view that to meet the priorities for palliative wound management provision of a moist wound environment is necessary and argue that this position does not represent an unrealistic attempt to heal 'non-healing wounds' (Bale, 1989; Gilchrist and Corner, 1989; Saunders and Regnard, 1989; Clark, 1992; Grocott, 1992c; Collinson, 1993; Miller *et al*, 1993; Fairburn, 1994).

The brief comparison (table 12.1) of the priorities for symptom control, the principle of moist wound healing, together with the characteristics of the 'ideal wound dressing', illustrates that theoretically the former supports the latter, with the proviso that systemic medications are included to overcome all the problems identified for these patients.

Table 12.1 Comparison of the priorities of symptom control

Priorities for Symptom Control at the Wound Site	The Principle of Moist Wound Healing/Characteristics of the 'Ideal Dressing'
• control of pain	• control of pain through maintenance of optimum humidity at the wound site (Thomas, 1989)
• prevention of complications e.g. infection, malodour, bleeding	• wound debridement with removal of excess exudate, toxic materials in order to prevent deterioration and control smell (Bale, 1989, Falanga 1988).
• control of exudate, including minimal disturbance to the patient because of frequent dressing changes	• the use of dressings which may remain *in situ* for 1–5 days. (Thomas, 1990; Collinson, 1993)
• removal of dressings without trauma	• dressing removal without trauma because the interface between the dressing and the wound is exudate (Gilchrist and Corner, 1989)
• restoration of body symmetry	• restoration of body symmetry through use of cavity dressings (Saunders and Regnard, 1989)
• cosmetic acceptability	• cosmetic acceptability when a primary dressing is adequate without the need for bulky secondary dressings (Saunders and Regnard, 1989); Grocott 1992a)

This theoretical approach to palliative wound management, however, has not been evaluated beyond a single-case study (Grocott, 1992b) and the case reports such as Collinson's (1993) and Boardman *et al* (1993). As well as data on incidence and location of fungating wounds, Thomas's (1992) survey revealed current practices in relation to the management of fungating lesions and radiation damaged skin and proposed a set of summary recommendations to assist in the formulation of guidelines for treatment. He also emphasised that the recommendations are not based on the results of clinically controlled trials as this information is simply not available. Miller *et al* (1993) make a plea at the end of their chapter on the nursing management of fungating wounds for the efficacy of such protocols to be demonstrated through the research process, as does Fairburn (1994).

Conclusions

The conclusions drawn were that a case for this research could be made on the basis of clinical significance in terms of physical and psychological distress and the limitations identified in the performance of dressings. It could not be made on the basis of reliable data indicating the magnitude of incidence. The common omission of the topic as a clearly defined priority for cancer and palliative care research was counterbalanced by the researcher's experiences of the problem. These were matched by case reports by other practitioners, the recent increase in interest in the topic in the nursing and medical literature as well as by support for the research from cancer and palliative care specialists. Evidence that the research has not been substantiated by others was conclusive.

Formulating the Research Questions

Formulation of the research questions from the literature and other sources of influence requires identification of gaps in knowledge which the study seeks to fill and makes explicit the focus of the inquiry (Miles and Huberman, 1984; Cormack and Benson, 1991). For this topic, three significant gaps were identified. First, it is evident from the background information on the development, presentation and treatment of fungating wounds that the experience of the wound is unique to the individual. It is also evident that this aspect has not been studied which suggests a need to elicit patient experiences. Secondly, there are commonalities among the symptoms identified for these wounds. Patients may gain from the application of the theoretical perspective of moist wound healing to the palliative management of non-healing wounds. However, this has not been evaluated formally. Thirdly, the circumstance of unresolved fungation, when the practitioner has to manage the wound predominantly with local measures, emphasises the role of wound dressings in symptom management. The experiences of other practitioners supported both the researcher's observations of limitations in the performance of dressings and identification of a need to explore alternative means of dressing these wounds, such as the concept of an individually moulded accessory.

The conceptual framework of the research, therefore, has the following dimensions: patients' experiences of the impact of fungating wounds; symptom control needs in relation to the wound; the performance of wound dressings (based on the principle of moist wound healing) with the addition of individually moulded accessories as local symptom control measures. The research questions develop logically from this framework (figure 12.1).

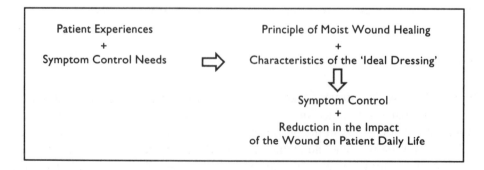

Figure 12.1   The conceptual framework

The Research Questions

• What are patients' experiences of the impact of a fungating malignant wound?
• How do wound dressings, which provide a moist wound environment, enhance symptom control and reduce the impact of the wound?
• How does the addition of an individually moulded wound support system enhance symptom control and reduce the impact of the wound?

The focus on the individual experience suggests the use of case studies as the overall research design (Yin, 1989; Stake, 1994). This, however, raises an epistemological question about the nature of knowledge generated from a single case and its value in clinical knowledge development. In this inquiry the intention is to reveal that the individual 'case' is both unique and complex. Across a population of 'cases' there are specific phenomena of interest in relation to recurring symptoms, dressing performance, professional time, dressing provision and costs. The inquiry will therefore extend to pattern identification from multiple cases with the potential for increasing understanding of the management of fungating wounds by making generalisations to theory in relation to the key concepts (Stake, 1994).

Endnote

The origins and motivation for conducting a research project into the palliative management of fungating wounds are in the individual experience of a nursing problem. As such it is a subjective view of the topic, the acknowledgement of which is a valued part of a disciplined inquiry. The contribution made by this chapter to a text on cancer and palliative care research lies in describing the preparatory work of moving the subject from the individual experience through to the justification of the study and the formulation of researchable questions.

References

Bale S (1989) Pressure sores in advanced disease: A flow diagram. *Palliative Medicine* 3(4):263–5.

Bale S and Harding K (1987) Fungating breast wounds. *Journal of District Nursing*, June, 4–5.

Banks V and Jones V (1993) Palliative care of a patient with terminal nasal carcinoma. *Journal of Wound Care* 2(1):14–15.

Bates T D (1984) Radiotherapy in Terminal Care. In: Saunders C (ed) *The Management of Terminal Malignant Disease*, 2nd edn. London: Edward Arnold.

Baum M, Breach N M, Shepard J H, Shearer R J, Meirion Thomas J and Ball A (1993)

Surgical palliation. In: Doyle D, Hanks G W and MacDonald N (eds) *Oxford Textbook of Palliative Medicine*. Oxford: Oxford University Press.

Bennett M (1985) As normal a life as possible. *Community Outlook*, February, 35–8.

Boardman M, Mellor K and Neville B (1993) Treating a patient with a heavily exuding malodorous fungating ulcer. *Journal of Wound Care* 2(2):74–6.

Bolton L and van Rijswijk L (1991) Wound dressings: Meeting clinical and biological needs. *Dermatology Nursing* 3(3):146–61.

Brennan S, Foster M E and Leaper D J (1986) Antiseptic toxicity in wound healing by secondary intention. *Journal of Hospital Infection* 8:263–7.

Brennan S, Levin V, Hacking A, Mills E, Gudgeon A, Bental N, Barry L, Creef L, Daniel V, Stannard C, Werner I D and Smit B J (1994) Neutron Irradiation in Locally Advanced Breast Carcinoma. *Neutrons in Cancer Therapy. Users' Results and Comments*. Report of the Neutrons in Cancer Therapy Conference, Cambridge 1992.

Bycroft L (1994) Care of a handicapped woman with metastatic breast cancer. *British Journal of Nursing* 3(3):126–33.

Chaplin D J (1992) Review: Chemical modifiers of blood flow. *Annual Report of the Cancer Research Campaign Gray Laboratory*. London: Cancer Research Campaign.

Clark L (1992) Caring for fungating tumours. *Nursing Times* 88(12):66–70.

Clinch J J and Schipper H (1993) Quality of Life Assessment in Palliative Care. In: Doyle D, Hanks G W and MacDonald N (eds) *Oxford Textbook of Palliative Medicine*. Oxford: Oxford University Press.

Collinson G P (1993) Fungating malignant wounds: Nursing management. *Wound Management* 4(2):54–5.

Copp G and Dunn V (1993) Frequent and difficult problems perceived by nurses caring for the dying in community, hospice and acute care settings. *Palliative Medicine* 7(1):19–25.

Cormack D F S and Benson D C (1991) Asking the Research Question. In: Cormack D F S (ed) *The Research Process in Nursing*. Oxford: Blackwell Scientific Publications.

Cutting K F and Harding K (1994) Criteria for identifying wound infection. *Journal of Wound Care* 3(4):198–201.

Deas J, Billings P, Brennan S, Silver I and Leaper D J (1986) The toxicity of commonly used antiseptics on fibroblasts in tissue culture. *Phlebology* 1:205–9.

Degner L (1987) Priorities for cancer nursing research: a Canadian replication. *Cancer Nursing* 10(6):319–26.

Doyle D (1987) *Domiciliary Terminal Care*. Edinburgh: Churchill Livingstone.

Doyle D, Hanks G and MacDonald N (1993) Introduction. In: Doyle D, Hanks G W and MacDonald N (eds) *Oxford Textbook of Palliative Medicine*. Oxford: Oxford University Press.

Fairburn K (1993) Towards better care for women: Understanding fungating breast lesions. *Professional Nurse* 8(12):204–12.

Fairburn K (1994) A challenge that requires further research: Management of fungating breast lesions. *Professional Nurse* 9(1):272–7.

Falanga V (1988) Occlusive wound dressings: Why, when, which? *Arch. Dermatol.* 124:872–7.

Fear M (1993) Addressing the problems of fungating wounds. *Primary Health Care* 3(1):18–21.

Finlay I (1991) The management of other frequently encountered symptoms. In: Penson J and Fisher R (eds) *Palliative Care for People with Cancer*. London: Edward Arnold.

Gilchrist B and Corner J (1989) Pressure Sores: prevention and management – A nursing perspective. *Palliative Medicine* 3(4):257–61.

Grant M M and Padilla G V (1983) An overview of cancer nursing research. *Oncology Nursing Forum* 10(1):58–67.

Grocott P (1992a) The latest on latex. *Nursing Times* 88(12):61–2.

Grocott P (1992b) *An Exploratory Study into the Use of a Foam Latex Support System for Ulcerating or Fungating Malignant Lesions: Patient, Family and Professional Experiences*. Unpublished BSc dissertation, King's College, University of London.

Grocott P (1992c) Application of the Principles of Modern Wound Management for Complex Wounds in Palliative Care. In: Harding K G, Leaper D L and Turner T D (eds) *Proceedings of the 1st European Conference on Advances in Wound Management*. London: Macmillan Magazines.

Grocott P (1993) Fungating malignant wounds. I: An overview and priorities for palliative management. *Wound management* 4(2):S2–S3.

Hanratty J R (1989) *Palliative Care of the Terminally Ill*. Oxford: Radcliffe Publications.

Higginson I and McCarthy M (1987) A prospective study of symptom control by a terminal care support team. In: Doyle D (ed) 1986 *International symposium on pain control. International Symposium Series* 123:81–6. London: Royal Society of Medicine.

Hirst D G (1992) Tumour Vascular Physiology. *Annual Report of the Cancer Research Campaign Gray Laboratory*. London: Cancer Research Campaign.

Hockley J M, Dunlop R and Davies R J (1988) Survey of distressing symptoms in dying patients and their families in hospital and the response to a symptom control team. *British Medical Journal* 296:1715–17.

Holmes S (1991) Preliminary investigations of symptom distress in two cancer patient populations: Evaluation of a measurement instrument. *Journal of Advanced Nursing* 16(4):439–46.

Hoskin P J (1993) Radiotherapy in Symptom Management. In: Doyle D, Hanks G W and MacDonald N (eds) *Oxford Textbook of Palliative Medicine*. Oxford: Oxford Medical Publications.

Hospice Information Service (1994) *Directory of Hospice and Palliative Care Services in the United Kingdom and Ireland*. London: Hospice Information Service at St Christopher's Hospice.

Hoy A (1993) Other Symptom Challenges. In: Saunders C and Sykes N (eds) *The Management of Terminal Malignant Disease*. London: Edward Arnold.

Humzah M D, Gazet J C and Ford H T (1992) Low Power Laser (LPL) Therapy in Malignant Ulcers. In: Harding K G, Leaper D L and Turner T D (eds) *Proceedings of the 1st European Conference on Advances in Wound Management*. London: Macmillan Magazines.

IHSM (1993) *Hospitals and Health Services Yearbook 1993*. London: Institute of Health Services Management.

Ivetic O (1991) *The Development and Diffusion of Wound Healing Theory and Practice: A Sociological Case-Study*. Unpublished PhD thesis, University of Sheffield.

Kearsley J H (1994) Some basic guidelines in the use of chemotherapy for patients with incurable malignancy. *Palliative Medicine* 4(1):11–17.

Lethem W (1993) Mouth and skin problems. In: Saunders C and Sykes N (eds) *The Management of Terminal Malignant Disease,* 3rd edn. London: Edward Arnold.

Lister A (1991) Care of patients with malignant wounds. *Wound Management* 1(3):13–15.

Love R R (1990) The Natural History of Cancer in Humans. In: Hossfield D K, Sherman C D, Love R R and Bosch F X (eds) *Manual of Clinical Oncology,* 5th edn. New York: Springer.

McCorkle R and Young K (1978) Development of a symptom distress scale. *Cancer Nursing* 1:373–8.

MacDonald N (1993a) Principles Governing the Use of Cancer Chemotherapy in Palliative Medicine. In: Doyle D, Hanks G W and MacDonald N (eds) *Oxford Textbook of Palliative Medicine.* Oxford: Oxford Medical Publications.

MacDonald N (1993b) The Interface between Oncology and Palliative Medicine. In: Doyle D, Hanks G W and MacDonald N (eds) *Oxford Textbook of Palliative Medicine.* Oxford: Oxford University Press.

McMahon R (1994) Trial and Error: An Experiment in Practice. In: Buckeldee J and McMahon R (eds) *The Research Experience in Nursing.* London: Chapman and Hall.

Miles M B and Huberman M A (1984) *Qualitative Data Analysis: A Source Book of New Methods.* Newbury Park, California: Sage.

Miller C, O'Neill A and Mortimer P (1993) Skin Problems in Palliative Care: Nursing Aspects. In: Doyle D, Hanks G W and MacDonald N (eds) *Oxford Textbook of Palliative Medicine.* Oxford: Oxford University Press.

Moody M and Grocott P (1993) Let us extend our knowledge base: Assessment and management of fungating wounds. *Professional Nurse* 8(9):586–90.

Mortimer P (1993) Skin Problems in Palliative Care: Medical Aspects. In: Doyle D, Hanks G W and MacDonald N (eds) *Oxford Textbook of Palliative Medicine.* Oxford: Oxford University Press.

Mosley J G (1988) *Palliation in Malignant Disease.* Edinburgh: Churchill Livingstone.

NACNEWS (1993) *Neutron Therapy Results at the National Accelerator Centre, April 1-2.* Faure, South Africa: National Accelerator Centre.

NCHSPCS (1993) *Evidence Submitted to the House of Commons Select Committee on Health Priority Setting in the NHS: The Drugs Budget on Extending the Drug Tariff.* London: National Council for Hospice and Specialist Palliative Care Services.

Neal K (1991) Treating fungating lesions. *Nursing Times* 87(23):84–5.

Nursing Times Editorial (1994) 90(31):8.

Oberst M (1978) Priorities in cancer nursing research. *Cancer Nursing* 1(4):281–90.

Preston K M and Griffen J (1989) Complex wound management: A case study. *Rehabilitation Nursing:* 14(5):269–70.

Regnard C F and Davies A (1986) *A Guide to Symptom Relief in Advanced Cancer,* 2nd edn. Manchester: Haigh and Hochland.

Regnard C F and Tempest S (1992) *A Guide to Symptom Relief in Advanced Cancer.* 3rd edn. Manchester: Haigh and Hochland.

Robbins J (ed) (1989) Nursing Care: Planning, Implementation and Evaluation. *Caring for the Dying Patient and the Family,* 2nd edn. London: Harper and Row.

Saunders J and Regnard C (1989) Management of malignant ulcers – A flow diagram. *Palliative Medicine* **3**(3):153–5.

Sims R and Fitzgerald V (1985) *Community Nursing Management of Patients with Ulcerating/Fungating Malignant Breast Disease.* London: Oncology Nursing Society.

Skolyszewski J, Korzeniowski S and Huckowski J (1994) Extensive Chest Wall Recurrence of Breast Cancer: A Possible Indication for Neutron Therapy. *Neutrons in Cancer Therapy. Users' Results and Comments.* Report of the Neutrons in Cancer Therapy Conference, Cambridge 1992.

Stake R E (1994) Case Studies. In: Denzin N K and Lincoln Y S (eds) *Handbook of Qualitative Research.* Newbury Park, California: Sage.

Stannard C, Hille J, Wilson J and Mills E (1994) Salivary Gland Myoepithelial Tumours. *Neutrons in Cancer Therapy. Users' Results and Comments.* Report of the Neutrons in Cancer Therapy Conference, Cambridge 1992.

Thomas M (1988) Coping with Distressing Symptoms. In: Wilson-Barnett J and Raiman J (eds) *Nursing Issues and Research in Terminal Care.* Chichester: John Wiley and Sons.

Thomas S (1989) Pain and wound management. *Nursing Times: Community Outlook* **85**:11–15.

Thomas S (1990) *Wound Management and Wound Dressings.* London: Pharmaceutical Press.

Thomas S (1992) *Current Practices in the Management of Fungating Lesions and Radiation Damaged Skin.* Bridgend, Mid Glamorgan: Surgical Materials Testing Laboratory.

Twycross R G and Lack S A (1990) *Therapeutics in Terminal Cancer,* 2nd edn. Edinburgh: Churchill Livingstone.

Vainio A (1991) WHO news. Prevalence of symptoms in cancer. *Palliative Medicine* **5**(4):275–6.

Walsh T D and West T S (1988) Controlling symptoms in advanced cancer. *British Medical Journal* **296**:477–81.

WHO (1990) *Cancer Pain Relief and Palliative Care.* Technical Report Series 804. Geneva: World Health Organisation.

Willis R A (1973) *The Spread of Tumours in the Human Body*, 3rd edn. London: Butterworth.

Wilson-Barnett J and Raiman J (eds) (1988) *Nursing Issues and Research in Terminal Care.* Chichester: John Wiley and Sons.

Wilson-Barnett J and Richardson A (1993) Nursing research and palliative care. In: Doyle D, Hanks G and MacDonald N (eds) *Oxford Textbook of Palliative Medicine.* Oxford: Oxford University Press.

Winter G D (1962) Formation of the scab and the rate of epithelialisation of superficial wounds in the skin of the young domestic pig. *Nature* **193**(4812):293–4.

Woodhouse P (1992) Managing a breast wound. *Nursing Times* **88**(12):72–5.

Yin R (1989) *Case Study Research. Design and Methods,* 2nd edn. Newbury Park, California: Sage.

Chapter 13
The Pattern of Fatigue in Patients Receiving Chemotherapy
Alison Richardson

Introduction

Of all the symptoms associated with cancer and its treatment, fatigue appears to be the most prevalent and also the most difficult for researchers to investigate. However, interest in this area is growing, fuelled by the recognition that fatigue is a phenomenon experienced by other client groups and worthy of systematic study (Potempa, 1993).

From the patients' perspective, fatigue has been reported as the most disturbing symptom experienced during treatment (Rhodes *et al*, 1988) with the greatest potential interference with self-care (Fernsler, 1986). Quality of life is affected profoundly as ability to perform household tasks and enjoy leisure activities becomes disrupted (Todres and Wojtuik, 1979), leading to impaired self-concept when roles and relationships are changed in consequence (Aistars, 1987).

There is clear evidence that fatigue is the most common side-effect for patients receiving chemotherapy. The occurrence of fatigue in cancer patients undergoing chemotherapy has been estimated. Coates *et al* (1983) surveyed a varied group of patients, asking them to identify and rank the physical and non-physical side-effects of chemotherapy. Experiencing constant tiredness was ranked highly overall, but its relative importance to other symptoms varied. Meyerowitz *et al* (1979), while outlining the psychosocial implications of adjuvant chemotherapy in breast cancer patients, reported fatigue in 96 per cent of the sample (*n*=50). It was described as the most common and disruptive symptom. Studies involving patients receiving chemotherapy for different types of cancer report the occurrence of fatigue as ranging from 59 per cent to 82 per cent of the sample (Nerenz *et al*, 1982; Cassileth *et al*, 1985; Nail and King, 1987; Nail *et al*, 1991). Fatigue has also been identified as the most distressing side-effect reported by patients receiving chemotherapy (Knobf, 1986; Strauman, 1986). Contradictory data regarding the intensity, frequency and level of distress culminating from fatigue associated with chemotherapy may be partially the result of conceptual and measurement differences among studies. Winningham *et al* (1994) point out that some researchers have asked patients whether they have experienced fatigue, while many have employed fatigue severity rating scales or sought information with symptom distress scales, combining information on the presence of fatigue and response to fatigue.

It is possible that fatigue may be caused by a number of factors in cancer patients. The exact mechanisms leading to fatigue remain to be established but several variables acting singly or in combination have been suggested as possibly contributing to it (Piper *et al*, 1987). Until a physiological basis has been discovered, it seems prudent to identify other factors which may contribute to the sensation of fatigue in this population. Studies should identify the intensity, duration, pattern and trajectory of fatigue and associated symptoms, and examine relationships between fatigue and demographic, disease-related and psychosocial correlates of fatigue. Such research would be valuable because it could initiate interventions aimed at the prevention and amelioration of fatigue.

Previous research reveals that patients often relate fatigue directly to treatment, the presence of other symptoms, degree of activity and psychological concerns (Piper, 1989). It appears to constitute an important problem regardless of cancer diagnosis and type of drug treatment, although the time of onset, duration, pattern, and severity of fatigue associated with chemotherapy and differences in the pattern of fatigue specific to individual drug combinations are not well described (Rhodes *et al*, 1988; Jamar, 1989; Pickard-Holley, 1991).

Rationale for the Study

Most studies concerned with fatigue in clinical populations have adopted cross-sectional research designs, and have sought to examine factors influencing fatigue. Consequently, the knowledge base from which to plan and initiate care is fragmentary, research neither confirming nor refuting previously accummulated results. A number of research studies undertaken with cancer chemotherapy patients have produced cross-sectional data at predetermined intervals (see Irvine *et al*, 1991 and Richardson, 1995). These do not take into account any pattern which may follow chemotherapy, but this should be an important consideration in the design of any study concerned with fatigue. Measures must be timed to document when fatigue develops in relationship to treatment; assumptions are often made about fatigue in the intervals between these measurements and an over-reliance on retrospective recall at interview is evident. Researchers risk missing important changes during intervals, including decline in health status which is later reversed. The present study sought to overcome some of these drawbacks, employing a research design which would record trends and changes over time.

The Study Design

The purpose of the study was to monitor the subjective dimensions of fatigue in patients receiving cytotoxic chemotherapy as a treatment for cancer, and to provide a description of the relationships of a number of factors postulated to influence this phenomenon. In addition, the researcher wished to document the nature of any interventions utilised by patients in response to fatigue and the effectiveness of such measures.

The study design was developed from a review of the literature considering previous methods of measurement, a decision supported by the researcher's extensive clinical experience with chemotherapy patients. It was refined through a series of pre-tests and a pilot study of the selected instruments and design. The longitudinal design involved the use of repeated measurements on the same individual, at daily and seven-day intervals to detect changes in individual patients and groups of patients over time. The research design and data collection schedules were chosen with an emphasis on minimising patient, staff and institutional burden. A schematic representation of the design is presented in figure 13.1.

Several key areas were explored in order to fulfil the purpose of the study. The researcher sought to:

• Monitor the subjective dimensions of fatigue (including information concerned with the onset, pattern, duration, intensity and distress caused by this phenomenon), as documented by the subjects in a daily diary designed by the researcher, and maintained over the period of 21–28 days following the administration of a pulse of chemotherapy;

• Describe the nature of the relationship between factors associated with fatigue in this patient population which may influence it, such as mood, as measured by the Mood Adjective Checklist (Lishman, 1972), symptom distress, as measured by the Holmes Symptom Distress Scale (Holmes, 1989), and a selection of demographic variables associated with this population, such as the type, pattern and nature of chemotherapy drugs received, stage of disease and type of cancer;

• Describe the self-care interventions which patients utilise in response to fatigue and the perceived effectiveness and source of ideas for such interventions.

• Test aspects of reliability and validity of the instruments used in the description of fatigue and the other variables, namely the Holmes Symptom Distress Scale, Mood Adjective Checklist, Fatigue Diary and the Piper Fatigue Scale (Piper *et al*, 1989).

This chapter will describe the methods employed to collect data on a daily basis through the use of the diary and the resulting findings.

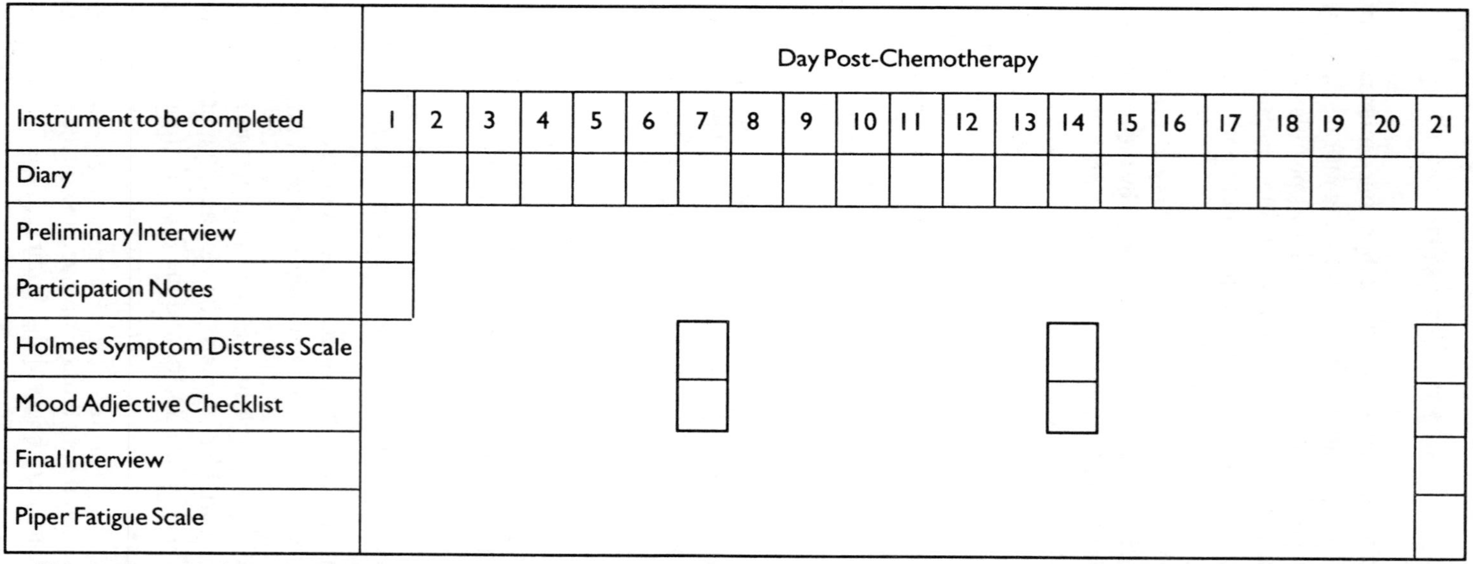

Instrument to be completed	1	2	3	4	5	6	7	8	9	10	11	12	13	14	15	16	17	18	19	20	21
									Day Post-Chemotherapy												
Diary																					
Preliminary Interview																					
Participation Notes																					
Holmes Symptom Distress Scale							☐							☐							☐
Mood Adjective Checklist							☐							☐							☐
Final Interview																					☐
Piper Fatigue Scale																					☐

This assumes a 21-day cycle of chemotherapy; data collection extends for those subjects receiving chemotherapy based on a 28-day cycle, at which point the final interview and Piper Fatigue Scale would be completed.

Day 1 is the day the patient receives chemotherapy.

Figure 13.1 Schematic representation of the design of the study

The Data Collection Instrument

The diary provided the means to elicit information concerning the daily differences in fatigue and a record of patient-initiated interventions performed to help the participant cope with fatigue during the previous 24 hours. It was envisaged that the diary would also yield data illustrating the development of interventions in relation to the experience of fatigue. In addition the diary was designed to record the experience of selected factors postulated to influence fatigue in cancer patients receiving chemotherapy on a daily basis. A review of the literature (Richardson, 1994a) suggested that, although diaries have not been used extensively in nursing research, the approach would be likely to yield valuable data when used with cancer patients (Richardson, 1994b).

Completion of the diary occurred on a daily basis for a pulse of chemotherapy (the exact number of days was dependent on the protocol the subject received). Each day the participant responded to items concerned with aspects of mood, symptoms, the selected dimensions of fatigue and self-care management strategies. The diary was divided into two parts, each consisting of a number of elements:

A. Six visual analogue scales exploring aspects of mood, appetite, sleep and nausea. These made up the first section.

B. Four visual analogue scales representing various dimensions of the fatigue experience, and boxes checked to confirm the presence of fatigue at specific times of day.

C. A record for patients to document any actions performed to relieve fatigue, their effectiveness (rated on a four-point scale) and the source of the idea. This portion of the diary was a self-report instrument adapted from the questionnaire and log of Dodd (1982; 1983) designed to elicit information concerning self-care actions taken by patients in a previous 24-hour period.

D. Open-ended items eliciting ideas about the contributory causes of fatigue and any symptoms experienced that day.

Elements B, C and D comprised the second section, and were completed if the respondent had experienced fatigue that day. Scoring of the diary was by measurement of each visual analogue scale, and a coding system was developed to record the presence or absence of fatigue at various times of day, performance of self-care behaviours and description of the open-ended responses.

Subjects for the research study were recruited from an oncology unit situated within a large London teaching hospital. The oncology unit comprised an inpatient facility of 26 beds and a variety of outpatient clinics. These facilities were served by a team of specialist doctors and nurses who catered for patients during the diagnostic, treatment and palliative stages of disease. Adjacent to the inpatient facility was situated the chemotherapy suite where patients would receive bolus and short-term infusional chemotherapy treatments. Initially it was planned to recruit a stratified convenience sample of approximately 90 patients comprising those with a diagnosis of small cell lung cancer, breast cancer, a gynaecological malignancy or a lymphoma, about to receive or in the process of receiving a course of chemotherapy. It was anticipated that this would lead to potential variation in the selected dimensions of fatigue and other influential variables to produce sufficient numbers to allow a statistical comparison. In practice, the researcher attempted to enrol a more diverse group of patients because a surgical consultant denied access to breast cancer patients. The population from which the sample was eventually drawn was expanded to include patients receiving chemotherapy of a continuous nature for gastrointestinal or pancreatic tumours. The characteristics of the sample are described in table 13.1.

Subjects were approached in the outpatient chemotherapy suite or the oncology ward at a time convenient to the patient and the multidisciplinary team. This was usually after a potential subject had received a bolus dose of chemotherapy or the continuous infusion had been newly primed.

Results

The patterns of change in the daily fatigue items recorded in the diary based on a visual analysis of the data will be detailed. Summary statistics of selected variables will also be presented.

Response Rate

One hundred and twenty-nine subjects consented to take part in the study. One hundred and nine subjects commenced the task of diary-keeping. Sixteen subjects failed to complete the diary. Five subjects died during the period of data collection and four of these diaries were not recovered. Major toxicity resulting in a period of hospitalisation or physical and/or mental deterioration which made it difficult for the subject to continue completing the diary resulted in the withdrawal of thirteen subjects at various time points (range 1–23 days). Nine subjects withdrew following consent after completing the diary for a variable number of days (range 2–16 days).

Themes

Each individual's time plots generated from the scores recorded on the visual analogue scales were reviewed for change. Mean fatigue time plots based on the

Table 13.1   Description of the sample *n* = 129

Age		Gender	
Mean	54 years	Male	44.2%
Range	26-82 years	Female	55.8%

Site of cancer		Time since diagnosis	
Ovary	20.16%	0 - 3 months	41.86%
Colorectal	15.50%	4 - 6 months	33.33%
Small Cell Lung	14.73%	7 - 12 months	8.53%
Non-Hodgkin's Lymphoma	13.95%	Over 12 months ago	16.28%
Gastric/Duodenum/ Oesophagus	13.18%		
Pancreas	5.43%	**Disease status prior to chemotherapy**	
Breast	5.43%	No disease	10.08%
Unknown Primary	4.65%	Locally advanced	32.56%
Hodgkin's Lymphoma	3.10%	Metastatic	57.36%
Bile Duct	2.33%		
Cervix	1.55%		

Treatment	
Carboplatin	20.16%
Epirubicin Cisplatin & 5-Fluorouracil (ECF)	20.16%
Epirubicin & Etoposide	14.73%
Cyclophosphamide, Epirubicin/Adriamycin, Vincristine & Prednisolone (CEOP/CHOP)	12.40%
5-Fluorouracil and Levamisole weekly	7.75%
Cyclophosphamide, Methotrexate and 5-Fluorouracil (CMF)	5.43%
Cisplatin and 5-Fluorouracil	5.43%
5-Fluorouracil weekly	5.43%
Chlorambucil, Procarbazine, Vinblastine, Prednisolone (CHLVPP)	2.33%
Continuous infusion of 5-Fluorouracil	2.33%
Cisplatin, Methotrexate and Bleomycin (PMB)	1.55%
Vincristine, Epirubicin, Etoposide and Prednisolone (VEEP)	1.55%
Etoposide, Ifosfamide, Cisplatin and Prednisolone (EPIC)	0.78%

Presence of Liver Metastases		Intended Outcome of Chemotherapy	
Negative	75.97%	Non-palliative	40.31%
Positive	24.03%	Palliative	59.69%

Purpose of Chemotherapy		Nature of Administration	
Neo Adjuvant	7.75%	Bolus and/or short term infusion	64.34%
Adjuvant	12.40%	Bolus and Continuous	20.16%
For Metastatic Disease	57.36%	Intermittent Bolus	13.18%
For Locally Advanced Disease	22.48%	Continuous	2.33%

Course		Previous Chemotherapy	
1	15.50%	Yes	13.18%
2	15.50%	No	86.82%
3	17.83%		
4	10.08%	**Previous Other Treatment**	
5	10.08%	Yes	42.64%
6	14.74%	No	57.36%
Not applicable	15.50%		

type of chemotherapy were generated for the aggregated data (see figure 13.2). A number of themes have been identified.

Mirror/parallel shifts
Shifts in the extent of fatigue on the visual analogue scale appear to be accompanied by corresponding shifts on the remaining scales concerned with the other dimensions of fatigue. As changes in the extent of fatigue occur they are closely mirrored by comparable changes in distress from fatigue and the level of interference from fatigue with daily activities/chores and enjoyable activities. The extent of fatigue rating appears to be persistently higher than the ratings of the other dimensions. There also appear to be parallel shifts in one or more of the visual analogue scales other than those concerned with fatigue. There is seldom a lag: the shifts occur in tandem on the same day.

Extensive declines and improvements
Increases in the extent of fatigue and the other dimensions tend to be considerable and abrupt, but decreases are typically gradual taking place over several days.

Stability versus dynamism
People tend to have one basic mode for the diary period: either persistently stable, perhaps with a couple of days on which levels obviously fluctuate, or moderately to highly dynamic. There is considerable diversity on every dimension.

Dynamics at start, middle and conclusion of diary
The administration of a bolus dose of chemotherapy often produces the most extreme mean fatigue value that an individual records during the diary period. For some, this occurs immediately following chemotherapy, and after a few days subsides. For the remainder this occurs a few days following administration. In those receiving traditional bolus/short-term infusion (CMF, Epirubicin and Etoposide, Carboplatin, CEOP, Cisplatin and 5-FU) or bolus plus a continuous infusion (ECF) there appears to be another abrupt increase in the mean fatigue score coinciding with the expected nadir, and again immediately before the next pulse. In people receiving weekly bolus injections of 5-FU a cyclical pattern is evident with increases in fatigue coinciding with the administration of chemotherapy. The degree of nausea recorded exhibits a different pattern. It is common for extreme scores to be achieved during the first few days and then gradually to decline throughout the rest of the week.

When the aggregated plots are inspected, it is possible to observe distinct patterns which are dependent on the type of chemotherapy received. Subjects receiving weekly chemotherapy (5-FU weekly and 5-FU and Levamisole) present a distinct and cyclical weekly pattern of fatigue. Those with metastases (the weekly 5-FU protocol) appear to attain higher mean fatigue scores compared to those receiving adjuvant therapy. Subjects receiving continuous plus bolus chemotherapy appear to reach a plateau value for fatigue ($\bar{X} \approx 20\text{--}30$), which appears to be

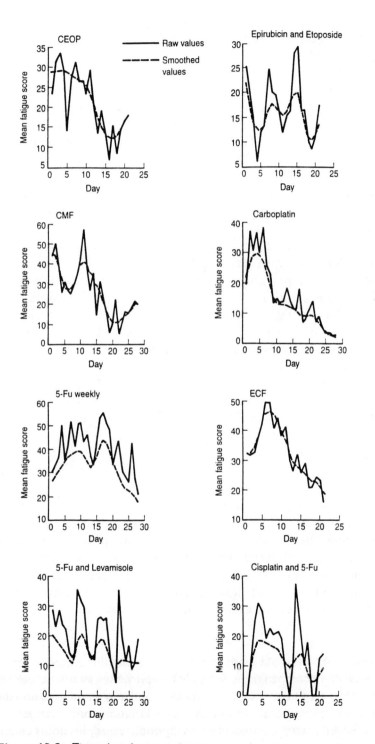

Figure 13.2   Time plots for mean fatigue scores by treatment protocol

greater than for those receiving conventional pulsed chemotherapy. For these subjects fatigue level appears to reach a peak at approximately an $\bar{X} \approx 30\text{–}45$ and then declines to a plateau between 0–20.

Subjects with breast cancer having CMF receive chemotherapy on day 1 and day 8 and take an oral drug on days 1–14. This is reflected in the pattern of fatigue: it remains relatively high for the first 14 days with a superimposed increase shortly after day 8. Subjects with a diagnosis of small cell lung cancer receiving the combination of Epirubicin and Etoposide appear not to be influenced by the fact that they continue to take oral Etoposide on days 1–4. Fatigue declines after day 1, rising again over days 5–7 and again at the expected nadir. It is pertinent to note that mean fatigue score rises sharply a few days prior to the next course of chemotherapy. This phenomenon also materialises in those subjects receiving CMF, CEOP and Cisplatin and 5-FU. The ovarian cancer subjects receiving single agent Carboplatin appear to experience fatigue during the first week post-infusion, but following this fatigue gradually declines, and during the fourth week reaches a particularly low level, probably indicating that the majority of this sample do not experience fatigue during the latter stage of the cycle. The Cisplatin and 5-FU regime for subjects with an unknown primary malignancy entails a five-day continuous infusion of 5-FU with Cisplatin administered over four hours on day 2. The mean fatigue scores remain raised during these five days with a gradual decline, followed around days 13–15 and days 20–21 by increases in fatigue. Non-Hodgkin's Lymphoma subjects receive bolus doses of chemotherapy on day 1 followed by a five-day course of oral Prednisolone. On the cessation of the Prednisolone there appears to be a rise in the level of fatigue.

Vignettes

Diary plots were created for all subjects who began the diary. The plots reproduced show the different trajectories for two subjects, using the raw data. The data were complex. In order to visualise them more easily and pick out trends a statistical transformation was performed. This is referred to as 'smoothing' the data. The plots in figures 13.3 and 13.4 are chosen to show different facets of change, some common and some not, and are accompanied by a commentary detailing the individual circumstances and experiences of these subjects.

Subject 1
Subject 1 was a 47-year-old woman with a diagnosis of metastatic breast cancer. She was receiving chemotherapy for palliative purposes as the cancer had spread to her liver. She had been diagnosed three months ago and was undergoing her third course of chemotherapy. Radiotherapy and surgery had not been attempted. She was widowed with two teenage sons who helped around the house with general tasks, but on the whole she coped independently with the cooking and

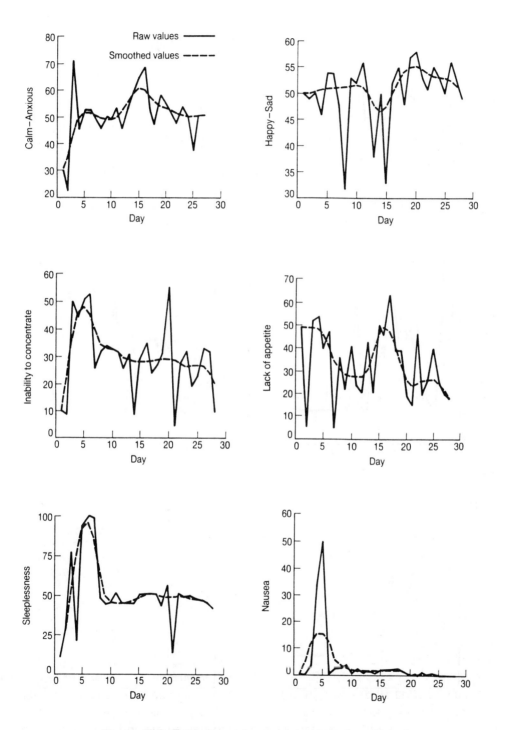

Figure 13.3 Time plots and summary statistics for subject 1
for each of the visual analogue scales

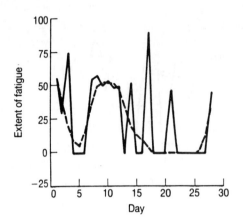

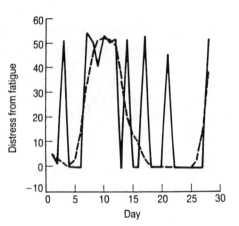

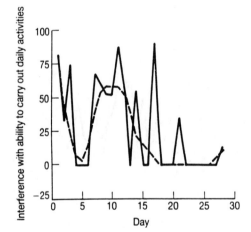

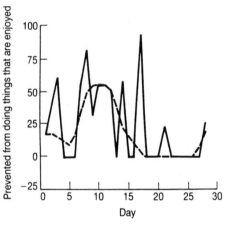

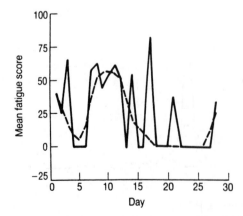

Summary statistics

Variable	Mean	Standard deviation
Calm–Anxious	50.58	10.44
Happy–Sad	50.11	6.36
Concentration	29.43	13.40
Appetite	33.07	15.37
Sleeplessness	50.54	21.57
Nausea	4.32	10.93
Extent	25.25	29.23
Distress	20.11	25.06
Daily activities	27.25	33.37
Hobbies	23.11	29.41
Mean FS	23.93	28.04

Figure 13.3 continued   Time plots and summary statistics for subject 1
for each of the visual analogue scales

cleaning. She found her job in full-time kitchen work too heavy to continue since the onset of her illness. This subject considered fatigue to be a worse sensation than tiredness and one that encompasses the whole body. She found fatigue to be a problem with the commencement of chemotherapy and attributed to the treatment poor sleep and the demands of looking after two teenage sons alone. She had not expected to feel fatigued but now expected it with every course. It occurred every day to some extent with a worsening on day 2 of the pulse, developing in the late afternoon and early evening.

The time plots of fatigue illustrate a fluctuating pattern, with the mean fatigue score ranging from 0–82 with an $\bar{X}$= 23.93 (S.D. = 28.04) and the subdimensions closely mirroring the mean fatigue score. As she had predicted, fatigue rose on day 2 and then disappeared for a number of days. Following this, fatigue exhibited a volatile pattern, severe on some days, completely absent on others. The other visual analogue scales seem to represent a parallel pattern apart from sleep and nausea. Nausea was only reported as a problem in the first week after which it subsided to become virtually absent, a common pattern in the majority of subjects. Problems with sleeping appeared to recur throughout the 28-day period, except for a slight improvement on day 21.

When she returned the diary to the researcher and was asked whether she had experienced any change in her health status during the past 28 days, she felt she had been more moody, and accounted for this by the fact that she was 'fighting' more with her sons. At home she felt she was managing more of the house. Fatigue had improved but she was unsure why, suggesting that the fact that spring appeared to be on the way might have accounted for this. She reflected that she had not done anything that had helped significantly to alter her fatigue, and indeed this was confirmed in the lack of recordings in the diary concerned with self-care actions, except on one day when she baked a cake with her small niece.

Subject 14

Subject 14 was a 61-year-old man who had been receiving weekly injections of 5-FU for colorectal cancer with multiple liver metastases for the last five months. The cancer had been diagnosed over six months ago when he underwent laparotomy and right hemicolectomy. He lives with his wife and between them they managed the daily chores, although he admitted that his wife took the main share because of his sciatica. He played an active role in the church and occasionally gave a sermon. He considered that tiredness and fatigue represented the same feelings. Fatigue had been a problem recently and he attributed this to treatment and expected it to be a continuing problem. He felt his present fatigue was the same as the fatigue he had encountered prior to his illness and that there was nothing abnormal or unusual about it. It occurred every day but not for all of the day, tending to coincide with the preaching pattern.

Fatigue fluctuated in a weekly cycle, tending to rise in the days following an injection of chemotherapy on days 1, 7, 13, and 21 and fall to zero just before the

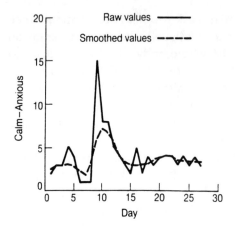

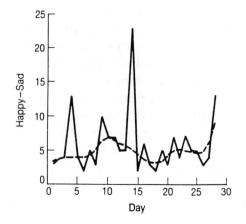

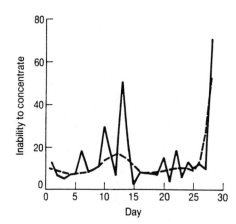

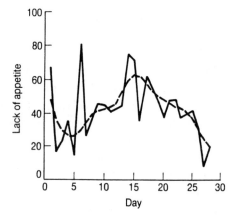

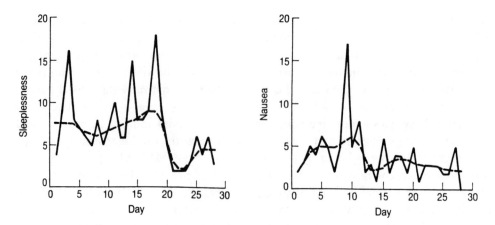

Figure 13.4 Time plots and summary statistics for subject 14
for each of the visual analogue scales

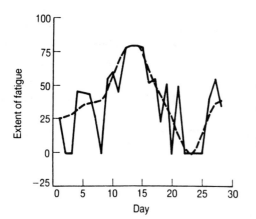

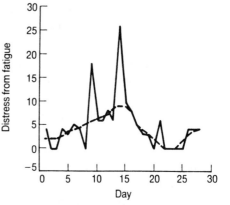

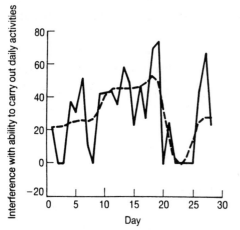

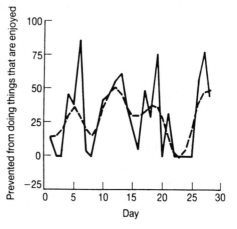

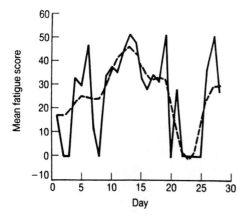

Summary statistics

Variable	Mean	Standard deviation
Calm–Anxious	4.17	2.89
Happy–Sad	5.86	4.41
Concentration	14.43	14.61
Appetite	42.39	17.85
Sleeplessness	7.04	4.00
Nausea	3.93	3.14
Extent	36.75	27.71
Distress	4.89	5.69
Daily activities	29.54	23.81
Hobbies	29.89	27.20
Mean FS	25.27	18.66

Figure 13.4 continued Time plots and summary statistics for subject 14 for each of the visual analogue scales

next injection. Diarrhoea was reported as a constant problem throughout the diary-keeping period as was pain due to sciatica, both worsening during the 7–21 day period. During days 7–21 fatigue remained relatively high, which was attributed to an increase in pain and a very busy period in terms of work which necessitated travelling long distances. The additional visual analogue scales depict a relatively calm and happy person little troubled by nausea or poor sleep, although a lack of appetite seemed to persist ($\bar{X}$= 42.39, S.D.= 17.85). This basic profile of clear episodes of fatigue following the administration of chemotherapy is typical of many subjects receiving weekly injections of 5-FU.

The subject felt his health status on the whole had remained stable during the data-collection period and things at home had been the same. He commented that his fatigue had not significantly altered and that it was caused by sciatica, a pre-existing health problem. When pressed on whether he had done anything that helped, he admitted that just sitting and resting in a chair with the occasional sleep during the day tended to dissipate his fatigue, although he did not record this in his diary.

Statistics also provide us with insight into the pattern of change and differences between groups. The richness of the individual daily data has at this point to be put aside for the sake of compact, objective summaries.

Aggregated Scores for Daily Diary Items

Eighty-nine per cent (98, total sample 109) of the sample reported fatigue at some point during the diary-keeping period, only 11 subjects failing to report any fatigue on any of their diary days. Figure 13.5 provides a graphic representation of the percentage of subjects experiencing fatigue on a daily basis over the diary-keeping period.

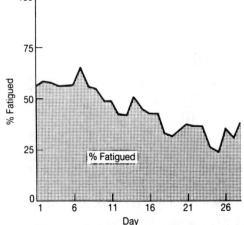

Figure 13.5 Percentage of patients experiencing fatigue on a daily basis

Subjects who experienced fatigue on a particular day were asked to indicate the periods of that day when they felt fatigued. Early afternoon, late afternoon and early evening appear to be the periods of day when the subjects are most likely to experience fatigue – 53.25 per cent ($n = 557$), 58.13 per cent ($n = 608$) and 57.27 per cent ($n = 599$) respectively, where n = number of observations rather than the number of individual subjects.

Table 13.2 describes the mean scores for items in the daily diary by the type of chemotherapy cycle the subjects were receiving. The mean fatigue scores for the 21-day, 28-day and weekly cycles are 25.94 (S.D. 23.2), 18.77 (S.D. 16.08) and 23.06 (26.37) respectively. These findings were significant ($H = 6.50$ 2 df $p = 0.039$). By considering the average ranks of the different groups, it was revealed that those subjects receiving a 21-day regime were significantly more fatigued than those undergoing either a 28-day or weekly regime.

Table 13.2 Mean scores of items in daily diary for subjects receiving a 21-day cycle, 28-day cycle and weekly cycle

Items in daily diary	21-day cycle (n=61)		28-day cycle (n=31)		Weekly cycle (n=17)	
	Mean	Standard deviation	Mean	Standard deviation	Mean	Standard deviation
Anxious-Calm	31.37	20.05	28.3	17.4	25.53	21.05
Happy-Sad	35.14	20.16	30.13	16.89	30.63	18.88
Ability to concentrate	34.02	17.06	27.52	17.86	32.6	24.39
Appetite	29.49	21.57	17.21	16.43	33.34	26.49
Sleep	35.84	21.33	28.6	16.9	30.52	22.2
Nausea	19.02	17.52	14.32	13.51	22.19	21.41
Extent of fatigue	29.08	25.33	23.69	19.09	24.18	25.91
Distress from fatigue	21.23	21.92	13.69	14.17	18.01	23.7
Interference with ability to carry out daily activities	25.9	23.87	18.8	17.45	24.56	28.59
Prevented from doing things that are enjoyed	26.98	25.17	18.69	16.09	25.49	29.02
Mean fatigue score	25.94	23.2	18.77	16.08	23.06	26.37

The data were examined using the Kruskal-Wallis test for comparing differences between groups, to see if there were any significant differences in the respondent mean fatigue scores in relation to the selected demographic variables. The significant results when differences in the mean fatigue score by selected demographic and medical variables were examined related to the site of the cancer ($H = 17.37$, 7 df, $p = 0.016$), type of chemotherapy ($H = 20.20$, 7 df, $p = 0.005$) and nature of administration ($H = 7.97$, 2 df, $p = 0.019$).

In relation to site of cancer, on examining the medians it appears that extent of fatigue is greater in those with a cholangiocarcinoma or pancreatic cancer, breast cancer or a lymphoma. Within the different types of chemotherapy those subjects receiving weekly 5-FU or ECF held the highest medians. The combination of bolus and continuous methods of administration resulted in higher fatigue scores.

Discussion

Together, the visual and statistical analyses confirm the dynamics in fatigue that cancer patients experience when being treated with chemotherapy. The current study supports and extends earlier research findings. Hence, clear progress in delineating the symptom has been made. This study has produced rich data and provides an advance over the lack of detail found in previous studies. Data which contain numerous repeated measurements have revealed distinct patterns of change and fluctuations. From the fine-grained data it is possible to gain a better idea about how often measurements should be taken. The approach to data collection facilitated the examination of relationships between the variables over consecutive days. This preserved the temporal relationships between the variables measured daily, which can be easily obscured when data are aggregated. The plots show how greatly people's trajectories of daily health may vary. The statistical analysis reveals the demographic and medical characteristics which influence the mean fatigue score.

The degree of fatigue and other dimensions selected for measurement in this study are related to the diagnosis and type of chemotherapy subjects received. The use of multivariate methods of analysis may make it possible to consider a model of factors which appear to influence fatigue in these groups. With the heterogeneity of the sample the sample size could be considered rather small, however, so this may not prove feasible.

The diary proved to be a useful means to track the selected variables and dimensions of fatigue. Missing data did inevitably lead to problems in conducting statistical analysis and as yet few guidelines are available in the literature as to how to handle such data.

The research approach required a great deal of flexibility and stamina on the part of the research team. The response rate and resilience of the subjects in completing the diary was positive. Some subjects refused to take part in the study and offered as an explanation for this that they did not wish to reflect on their circumstances over a protracted period of time. The desire to maintain a non-cancer identity was strong in these subjects, in essence leaving their cancer at the hospital, separating the role of chemotherapy patient from other roles they may have occupied. Talking in an interview might have been more acceptable for these subjects.

Escalation of physical and mental problems did undoubtedly lead subjects to quit the task of diary-keeping. Subjects sometimes remarked when they returned the diary that someone else had helped them, especially if there had been a few days when their health had deteriorated. Clarridge and Massagli (1989) refer to this as proxy reporting. Fayers and Jones (1983) point out that if the assessor is a close relative of the patient and is responsible for reporting on the patient's quality of life, problems may result from a confounding of the patient's view with the views of the observer. The use of other people to report symptoms when symptom levels escalate has been infrequently addressed, but this is precisely the time when measurements are needed and the patient is most unlikely to provide them.

The diary training was judged to be vital. It was particularly valuable for those subjects who remained in hospital for a few days to receive chemotherapy. These subjects were able to meet with the researcher, reviewing the diary completion and correcting any mistakes. This was more difficult by telephone, particularly if there was a problem in completing the visual analogue scales. The validity and reliability of this method of measuring fatigue will become clearer when the other parts of the study are analysed and the findings considered.

The fact that there is no contrast group of subjects could be viewed as a limitation of the study; differences in fatigue could not be definitively attributed to cancer and its treatment. The validity of comparing a healthy group whose feelings of fatigue are most likely to be associated with a hard day's work with the fatigue associated with a chronic illness could be questioned. An intimation that the quality and quantity of such fatigue is indeed different was given by the subjects when the question was posed during the interview. More open interviewing may reveal this, particularly if conducted over time and continuing into the period following the cessation of treatment.

Larger samples are required to confirm similarities and differences. In-depth interviewing about the fatigue experience is needed to clarify the multiple manifestations and meanings of fatigue. We must continue to describe the patient characteristics that are correlated with fatigue and assess the impact on people's lives. Further longitudinal, correlational and comparative studies will facilitate the examination of causal relationships. The lengthy and changing nature of a chronic illness such as cancer and its treatment add to the difficulty in developing a full picture of this phenomenon.

Clinical research is beginning to provide practitioners with information about the fatigue experience which can be used in clinical practice. These findings are important, as they provide an empirical base for guiding further research and practice. Nurses can use this information to warn patients of impending fatigue. Coaching well in advance of the anticipated problem and enabling the mobilisation of resources to help cope with fatigue could be beneficial. The importance of individualising any intervention based on the patient's fatigue experience should be recognised in any future intervention studies.

References

Aistars J (1987) Fatigue in the cancer patient: A conceptual approach to a clinical problem. *Oncology Nursing Forum* **14**(6):25–30.

Cassileth B, Lusk E, Bodenheimer B, Farber J, Jochimsen P and Morrin-Taylor B (1985) Chemotherapeutic toxicity – The relationship between patients' pre-treatment expectations and the post-treatment results. *American Journal of Clinical Oncology* **8**:419–25.

Clarridge B and Massagli M (1989) The use of female spouse proxies in common symptom reporting. *Medical Care* **27**(4):352–66.

Coates A, Abraham S, Kaye S, Sowerbutts T, Frewin C, Fox R and Tattersall M (1983) On the receiving end – Patient perception of the side-effects of cancer chemotherapy. *European Journal of Cancer and Clinical Oncology* **19**(2):203–8.

Dodd M (1982) Assessing patients' self-care for side-effects of cancer chemotherapy. *Cancer Nursing* **5**(6):447–51.

Dodd M (1983) Self-care for side-effects in cancer chemotherapy: An assessment of nursing interventions. *Cancer Nursing* **6**(1):63–7.

Fayers P and Jones D (1983) Measuring and analysing quality of life in cancer clinical trials: A review. *Statistics in Medicine* **2**:429–46.

Fernsler J (1986) A comparison of patient and nurse perceptions of patients' self-care deficits associated with cancer chemotherapy. *Cancer Nursing* **9**(2):50–7.

Holmes S (1989) Use of a modified symptom distress scale in assessment of the cancer patient. *International Journal of Nursing Studies* **26**(1):69–79.

Irvine D, Vincent L, Bubela N, Thompson L and Graydon J (1991) A critical appraisal of the research literature investigating fatigue in the individual with cancer. *Cancer Nursing* **14**(4):188–99.

Jamar S (1989) Fatigue in Women Receiving Chemotherapy for Ovarian Cancer. In: Funk S, Tornquist E, Champagne M, Archer Copp L and Wiese R (eds) *Key Aspects of Comfort: Management of Pain, Fatigue and Nausea.* New York: Springer.

Knobf M (1986) Physical and psychological distress associated with adjuvant chemotherapy in women with breast cancer. *Journal of Clinical Oncology* **4**(5):678–84.

Lishman W (1972) Selective factors in memory. Part 2: Affective disorders. *Psychological Medicine* **2**:248–53.

Meyerowitz B, Sparks F and Spears I (1979) Adjuvant chemotherapy for breast carcinoma: Psychosocial implications. *Cancer* **43**:1613–18.

Nail L, Jones L, Greene D, Schipper D and Jensen R (1991) Use and perceived efficacy of self-care activities in patients receiving chemotherapy. *Oncology Nursing Forum* **18**(5):883–7.

Nail L and King K (1987) Fatigue: A side-effect of cancer treatments. *Seminars in Oncology Nursing* **3**(4):257–62

Nerenz D, Leventhal H and Love R (1982) Factors contributing to emotional distress during cancer chemotherapy. *Cancer* **50**:1020–7.

Pickard-Holley S (1991) Fatigue in cancer patients – A descriptive study. *Cancer Nursing* **14**(1):13–19.

Piper B (1989) Fatigue: Current Bases for Practice. In: Funk S, Tornquist E, Champagne

M, Archer Copp L and Wiese R (eds) *Key Aspects of Comfort: Management of Pain, Fatigue and Nausea.* New York: Springer.

Piper B, Lindsey A and Dodd M (1987) Fatigue mechanisms in cancer patients: Developing a nursing theory. *Oncology Nursing Forum* **14**(6):17–23.

Piper B, Lindsey A, Dodd M, Ferketich S, Paul S and Weller S (1989) The Development of an Instrument to Measure the Subjective Dimension of Fatigue. In: Funk S, Tornquist E, Champagne M, Archer Copp L and Wiese R (eds) *Key Aspects of Comfort: Management of Pain, Fatigue and Nausea.* New York: Springer.

Potempa K (1993) Chronic Fatigue. In: Fitzpatrick J and Stevenson J (eds) *Annual Review of Nursing Research.* New York: Springer.

Rhodes V, Watson P and Hanson B (1988) Patients' descriptions of the influence of tiredness and weakness on self-care abilities. *Cancer Nursing* **11**(3):186–94.

Richardson A (1994a) The health diary: An example of its use as a data collection method. *Journal of Advanced Nursing* **19**:782–91.

Richardson A (1994b) Piloting a Study. In: Buckeldee J and McMahon R (eds) *The Research Experience in Nursing.* London: Chapman and Hall.

Richardson A (1995) Fatigue in cancer patients: A review of the literature. *European Journal of Cancer Care* **4**(1):20–32.

Strauman J (1986) Symptom distress in patients receiving phase 1 chemotherapy with Taxol. *Oncology Nursing Forum* **13**(5):40–3.

Todres R and Wojtuik R (1979) The cancer patient's view of chemotherapy. *Cancer Nursing* **2**(4):283–6.

Winningham M, Nail L, Barton Burke M, Brophy L, Cimprich B, Jones L, Pickard-Holley S, Rhodes V, St Pierre B, Beck S, Glass E, Mock V, Mooney K and Piper B (1994) Fatigue and the cancer experience: The state of the knowledge. *Oncology Nursing Forum* **21**(1):23–36.

Chapter 14
Progress to Date
Jenifer Wilson-Barnett

An exciting range of studies has been collected in this volume, emerging from what appears to be a genuine quest by researchers for understanding and solutions. These contributors are all active researchers wedded to the cancer and palliative nursing care field. Their accounts demonstrate commitment to nursing, but tend also to exploit other disciplines and hopefully benefit and possibly influence them. Topics chosen and methods selected to explore these, while being central to the practice and organisation of nursing, relate to established themes within psychology, sociology and human biology. Authors seem to have achieved mastery of both contributory disciplines and nursing.

Selection of these studies was based on the editors' knowledge of ongoing work across the country. As our aim was to encourage researchers to discuss their studies, whether completed or not, we were not over-selective. As the volume of this type of research work increases each year, this task was made easier. Fellowships and lectureships among cancer and palliative care researchers and nurses in particular have helped to develop a thriving network, where many have been fortunate enough to benefit from sponsorship or support from Cancer Relief Macmillan Fund. Without this impetus and healthy encouragement, this area of specialist research could not boast so many studies of such high quality.

Through a review of the preceding chapters, several themes emerge. The balance of research across the five years, in areas such as communications and emotional needs or aspects of physical care, remains unaltered. Perhaps the overwhelming importance of psychological support provided by nurses explains the popularity of this area. Only two studies explored physical problems representing the relative difficulties with this type of work, both intellectually and practically. Yet still there is abundant need to prevent unnecessary and extremely distressing symptoms and side-effects. Interestingly, here fewer studies focused on the organisation of care, across the team, whereas this was a dominant research theme in the previous five years. One hesitates to explain this as due to a successful resolution of organisational problems, as many of the current projects touch on this area as affecting delivery of care without concentrating on team work or continuity of care. Encouraging is the orientation to family welfare, at last showing that patients cannot be seen in isolation, as so much of what happens to them and influences their lives affects their relatives and significant others.

One of the most striking features of these studies is the desire by researchers to ask meaningful questions, not just complete a good piece of research. Maturity will come to the nursing discipline when the questions lead the research approach in this way. So many in the past may have been discouraged by ideas that their topic was 'not researchable' as appropriate methods did not exist. With tact, skill and imagination, these contributors ask searching and sensitive questions and have succeeded in producing some significant insights.

Recognition that most 'events' are determined by a plurality of factors means that measurement needs to reflect this. Continual questioning of previous work and the requirement to improve methods used in the past has forced research to create new tools, combine these with others and adopt an eclectic approach, searching for the most illuminating process.

Contributors have not been satisfied to do work which is removed from reality or which produces peripheral information, and emergent questions demonstrate this. Every single study has important implications for everyday practice, including, for instance: 'Why are ethnic minorities treated so indifferently? How can we change the service and professional prejudice? How can the appalling ignorance, self-confessed by staff, of cancer in elderly people be addressed? Does this reflect the attitude that somehow pervades society that the elderly and impoverished or immigrant groups do not require better care? Or is it amenable to educational input?

Other similar, fundamental questions emerge from these studies. Is the level of grief experienced in response to early diagnosis inevitable, or can it be buffered by improved communication and support? Given that nurses are aware that they are likely to face emotional disclosures as a consequence of open communication styles, how can we support them to retain this expertise and the necessary personal resources?

So many of these questions are now grounded in more established evidence. Just as the associated studies were so well grounded in previous work, future research must tease out ways of answering this next set of questions. Many of the conundrums presented in this way are central to health care practice and can be seen as major issues requiring substantial involvement of resources. Yet if public support is manifest nurses are in a good position to evaluate such changes.

Interestingly, much of the work contained in this book precedes or reflects the sentiments directing the NHS reforms and associated Department of Health *Strategy for Nursing Research* of 1993. Nursing theorists have long since advocated partnership, empowerment of clients and real choice. Several studies demonstrate the close involvement of researchers with participants in an attempt to share their perspectives or really explore the possibilities of more decision-making by recipients. Complex situations rarely reveal singular approaches, involvement in decision-making and care plans seems desirable to some, not all, and sensitivity in providing an arena where this is possible is easier in some contexts. Palliative care in particular has been held up by these editors previously as a forerunner and exemplar to others. Cancer care in contrast seems, from findings in these chapters, to require much more reorientation. Deprofessionalising health care needs to occur in a way which retains so much of what respondents appreciate, but abandons ill-considered approaches to consultation and care delivery.

Just as the government policy for cancer and palliative care is being more explicitly formulated by the Chief Medical Officer in the Calman Report (1994) with a more systematic distribution of services and specialist expertise, parallel plans need to be envisaged for nursing. The scale of the required services is now acknowledged to be greater than presently provided, and for nursing it is perhaps the balance between specialists and generalists and the associated skill levels which need review.

This nursing research epitomises the great differences revealed between specialist practice and generalist nursing care. Over the last decade this has been noted and discussed in research literature (see Wilson-Barnett and Raiman, 1988), but seemingly little has occurred to promote more integrated specialist practice or improved general hospital and community care for those with cancer or terminal illness. Contrasting pictures have been drawn by these researchers, for instance families with a child suffering cancer seemed to praise the expertise and support given by the paediatric cancer nurse specialists, and nurses in a dedicated hospital setting revealed a deep level of understanding of their own and their patients' psychological needs. This highlights the often unrecognised traumas of patients under the generalists' teams, awaiting diagnosis, responding to diagnosis or coping with apparently uncaring staff attitudes. Lack of knowledge and understanding rather than of altruism probably explains these inadequacies, and the scale of government reforms acknowledges this vast challenge. However, the requisite shift in attitudes and resources should not be allowed to denude general services. Increasingly it can be seen that research in a specialist area can be exploited in order to change general practice. Dissemination of good examples and of revelations with relevance to all nurses can be very helpful. Indeed, cancer and palliative care nurses have demonstrated expertise which should be shared with others in general nurse education and practice.

Pleas for more rational expenditure in the Health Service have encouraged evaluations of interventions and innovations. Specialist nurses themselves have not felt exempt from the need to provide evidence of their value. Studies with breast care nurses and Macmillan nurse tutors fall under this rubric. What seems to be revealed in these very different studies is the sheer commitment to their work and the deep concern about how their contribution could be improved. Tutors have so much to overcome at present with the dual reformations of the Health Service and Nursing Education. Their relative isolation is compounded by a divided loyalty to service and their educational institution. Hopefully in future this will be less of an issue, with more practitioners achieving their rightful role as educators and lecturers become much more oriented to service needs. Breast care specialists also echo this concern that they feel marginal to the main care team and often find it very difficult to form networks and establish working partnerships.

Isolation, therefore, is a problem for specialists and the associated stress of cancer and palliative care requires effective support systems. Many pathfinders in health care and researchers share this feeling of isolation, but benefit from colleague support, often in the form of peer-group discussions. Unless Macmillan nurses and others in similar positions receive this support, their contribution and level of expertise may deteriorate. Managers may be able to help in facilitating such support mechanisms or be personally involved in providing them. Alternatively or in conjunction the multidisciplinary team may be able to provide opportunities to share similar experiences and challenges. Meaningful continuing education, sabbatical leave with exchange of roles and mentorship arrangements are also required. Policy decisions are called for, as it may be necessary to redirect resources away from generating new posts (always popular with locality fund raisers) to programmes of support for more established experts who need succour and refreshment.

Just as the researchers have shown their willingness to become close to participants and feel emotionally drained by some of their discussions, so for practitioners it must be equally if not more stressful. Enduring strategies are required for both roles but, in order to provide genuine care, staff need skill and recognised, systematic support. Support groups have been set up in some academic departments for researchers. Many more are required for hospital, hospice and most importantly for community staff, who may become particularly isolated.

In many ways the trends noted in this collection of studies indicate a new level of maturity for this research and specialty. The sophisticated understanding demonstrated by so many of the authors provides encouraging thoughts for the future. Rigorous research and a very professional level of presentation are evident. Many have been supported by other researchers, senior academics in nursing or allied fields, and this has undoubtedly helped the outcome of these studies. However, it is the courage of researchers in tackling such difficult, emotive and distressing areas of care that is so valuable. Questioning those with a new diagnosis of cancer or providing an innovative method for dressing suppurating wounds are equally challenging and courageous. They typify the 'new nursing research ethos' – the issue or problem determines what study is required and nothing is beyond some imaginative person's brief.

In future, research which continues to address problems in patient and relative care, which reflects nursing concerns and which provides evidence for practice must build on what has gone before. Evaluations of new approaches to nursing care will probably be indicated if readers reflect or adopt the challenges raised by questions such as those in the middle of this chapter; without advocating mechanistic and wholly quantified measuring approaches, it would seem appropriate to assess changes and their effects methodically.

Combined methods can be illuminating and also laborious, but more meaningful results may ensue. Painstaking work by Richardson on fatigue demonstrated that repeated measurement could provide real insights into patients' responses. Data collection and analysis take a great deal of intelligence but more than all else tenacious application and dedication. This work then provides as much for future researchers as it does for practice. Clearly, guidelines for practice and education can be produced only after rigorous testing of tools and suggestions for improvements. In order to achieve truly research-based practice more of this is required. However, a variety of approaches and levels of research in exploration, description, interpretation and testing must be recognised and will inevitably be undertaken. Different types of research will have different effects on those who read it. Description may provoke thought and self-initiated changes, whereas systematic evaluation may be taken up at management level and lead to policy changes.

This specialty is one of the most advanced and well-supported, volumes such as this one hopefully reflecting this. As editors we are indebted to all the contributors who responded in a willing and typically positive way to our request for them to do yet more work. It is our profound hope that they will stimulate others and give them a sense of belonging to an energetic, intensely motivated and caring academic and practice-based discipline.

References

Calman Report (1994) *Policy Framework for Commissioning Cancer Services*. London: HMSO.

DoH (1994) *Report of the Taskforce on the Strategy for Research in Nursing, Midwifery and Health Visiting*. London: HMSO.

Wilson-Barnett J and Raiman J (1988) *Nursing Issues and Research in Terminal Care*. Chichester: John Wiley and Sons.

Index

alexithymia 180
alopecia, review of research (1989–1994)
    13, 15
anxiety, *see* Hospital Anxiety and
        Depression Scale
assessment, *see* needs; services
awareness
    of early warning signs 114, 126–7, 128
    lack of, as constraint on screening 118,
        120
    in older adults 126–9

bereavement
    models of 152
    and palliative care staff 151–2, 159–63
black and minority ethnic groups
    cancer rates in 85
    communication with 87–8, 92
    dietary requirements 90–1
    ethnic monitoring in NHS 85
    family and community networks 92–3
    information for 88, 89–90, 92, 93
    language problems 92
    and palliative care services 83–5,
        85–6
    racism 91, 94
    religious requirements 90–1
    service access 89–90
    support services 92–3

underuse of hospices 85–6
underutilisation of services 83, 84–5
unequal access to services 84, 93–4
use of term 83
black and minority ethnic groups and
        palliative care services, research study
    background 84–6
    discussion 91–4
    interviews 86
    language and communication 87–8
    methods 86
    population 84, 86
    results 86–91
    sample 86–7
blocking behaviours 171–2
    review of research (1989–1994) 8, 9
breast cancer
    changes in management of 189–90
    check-up guidelines 119
    clinical practice 108
    government target 104, 107
    incidence 27
    information, women's need for 201–2
    information sources 200
    minimisation of disease 201
    mortality rates 107, 189
    National Breast Screening Programme
        107–8, 189–90
    prevention a 'forgotten area' 118

previous studies 190
psychological consequences of 189
support needs for patients 27
see also breast screening; psychological
    morbidity
breast care nurses
    autonomy valued 36
    cancer nursing 40
    clinical nurse specialism 29, 40–1
    community liaison 39–40
    continuing need for 28
    counselling 39
    dimensions of care 37-8
    education and training 30, 38, 40, 41–2,
        43–4
    empowerment of patients 37–8
    frameworks for care 39
    holistic care 37
    increase in numbers of 28
    and job satisfaction 30, 34, 41–2
    need for focus on cancer nursing 42
    need for organizational developments 44
    networking 38
    nursing process 39
    nursing records 40, 44
    and patients' emotional problems 39,
        42
    and patients' spiritual needs 39, 41, 42
    personality differences 30, 33, 41
    psychological help to patients 28, 41
    RCN job description 29, 38
    and research-based practice 29–30, 41
    role background 27
    role evaluation 28
    role of 35–6
    social factors affecting 31
    standard setting 36–7
    suitability for job 30
breast care nurses, research study
    aims 29
    conclusions 42–3
    design 31–5
    inclusion criteria 32
    interviews 33
    methods 33
    population 32
    qualitative data analysis 34
    rationale 28–9
    recommendations 43-5
    results 35–42
    sample 32–3
    statistical analysis 35
    timing 34–5
Breast Care Nursing Society 29, 38
breast screening
    aim of 190
    National Breast Screening Programme
        107–8, 189–90
    reduced mortality 190
    reduced number of mastectomies 200
breast self-examination (BSE) 190

cancer
    anticipated increase in cases 113
    causes 126
    common types of 98
    early diagnosis and treatment 99
    emotional responses to 169–70
    fear of 127, 129, 130
    lack of ethnic data 85
    mortality 98, 99
    patients' experience of, review of
        research (1989–1994) 9–11
    predominantly in elderly 99
    registration 98, 105
    society's distorted image of 129
    see also awareness; early detection;
        health checks; prevention; screening;
        and specific cancers
cancer nurses
    blocking own skills? 177, 182
    communication skills 181–2
    feelings and anxieties 181–3
    helping role 167
    oncology education 103
    and patients' emotions 167–8
    role of, reports and recommendations
        102–3
Cancer Relief Macmillan Fund (CRMF)
    Breast Cancer Campaign 28
    funding of Macmillan Nurse Tutor posts
        49, 64

funding of POONS posts 68
see also Macmillan nurses
cancer services
    access to 100
    demand for 98
    development of policy 98–9
    government initiatives 104–10
    health checks 118, 119
    organisation of 103–4
    resource availability 101–2
    standards of care 100–1
    see also hospices; nurses; palliative care;
        screening cervical cancer
    check-up guidelines 119
    government target 104, 108
    mortality rates 108
    prevention a 'forgotten area' 118
    screening 108
chemotherapy
    reports and recommendations 101–2
    see also fatigue
children
    cancer treatment 70–1
    effect of prolonged hospitalisation 67
    effect on families of cancer in 70–1
    home care 67–8
    improvement in cancer treatments 67–8
    see also Paediatric Oncology Outreach
        Nurse Specialists
clinical nurse specialist (CNS) role in breast
    care nursing 29, 40–1
colleges of nursing
    changing values and priorities 56–8
    course evaluation 59–60
    enlargement and amalgamation 56
    impersonality of 61–2
    income generation 57–8, 63
    market-led reforms 61–2
    responsiveness to purchasers 59
    'sausage machines' 61–3
    surfeit of change 62–3
    see also education and training
colorectal cancer, check-up guidelines 119
communication
    with black and minority ethnic groups
        87–8, 92

cancer nurses' skills 181–2
    in framework of care 39
    nurses', review of research (1989–1994)
        8, 9
    training 183
community services, lack of childhood
    cancer expertise 68, 70–1, 73
counselling, by breast care nurses 39
CRMF, *see* Cancer Relief Macmillan Fund

death, professional *v.* personal management
    152
depression, *see* Hospital Anxiety and
    Depression Scale
detection, *see* early detection
DHAs, *see* District Health Authorities
diet, black and minority ethnic groups 90–1
disclosures, *see* emotional disclosures
distress
    with fungating malignant wounds
        210–12
    review of research (1989–1994) 9–12
    see also psychological morbidity
distress scales, review of research
    (1989–1994) 10, 11, 12
District Health Authorities (DHAs),
    responsibilities of 97
dressings 210–12, 215–16, 218

EAGC (Expert Advisory Group on Cancer)
    report 100, 100–1, 102, 103, 110
early detection of cancer in older adults
    constraints in primary health care
        117–22
    health checks 118
    strategies for 114
    see also awareness; screening; symptoms
        and signs
early detection of cancer in older adults,
    research study
    background 114–15
    conclusions 129–30
    design and methods 115–17
    interviews 116
    main emergent themes 117
    purpose 113

research questions 115
results and discussion 117–29
sample 115–16, 123
single case study 116–17
education and training
    breast care nurses 30, 38, 40, 41–2, 43–4
    cancer nurses 103
    cancer prevention training for nurses
        120
    changes in 249–50
    chemotherapy use 102
    communication skills 183
    detrimental effect on palliative care? 60
    hospice commitment to 54, 55
    institutional culture 56–63
    move towards specialist teachers 49–50
    Post-Registration Education and Practice
        49
    Project 2000 49, 56
    recent reforms and proposals 49
    responsibility for funding 60–1
    taking cervical smears 108
    see also colleges of nursing; Macmillan
        Nurse Tutors
elderly, see older adults
emotional disclosures
    alexithymia 180
    blocking behaviours 171–2
    and cancer 169–70, 180–1
    consequences of, on nurses 177–8
    cultural and social influences 168
    emotions felt v. emotions described
        168
    facilitating behaviours 171–2
    metaphor use 181
    method of making sense of experience
        169, 180–1
    nurses' avoidance of involvement
        170–1
    overt and covert 176–7, 180
    verbal strategies during 172–8
    voluntary control of 168
emotional disclosures, research study
    aims 172
    analysis of evidence 172–8
    conclusions 183

disclosive sequences 172–3, 174
discussion 178–83
method 169, 172
transcription notation 183–4
emotional labour 77
emotions
    denial of 170
    management 170
    in social context 168
empowerment, of patients by breast care
    nurses 37–8
English National Board (ENB)
    breast care nursing course 38
    and teacher specialisation 49
ethnic minority groups, see black and
    minority ethnic groups
ethnography 31
Expert Advisory Group on Cancer
    (EAGC) report 100, 100–1, 102,
    103, 110

face
    definition 178
    positive and negative 178
face-work 178, 179, 181–2, 183
facilitating behaviours 171–2
    review of research (1989–1994) 8, 9
families
    hospice as family 155–6
    hospice care for 158
    see also children
families, of newly diagnosed patients
    burden of illness 146–7
    coping methods 142–6
    different perceptions, families' and
        patients' 137
    lack of contact with health professionals
        148–9
    monitoring the patient 148
    non-disclosure 145–6
    and patients' activities 147–8
    patients' methods of coping 146
    prospect of death 143–4
    protecting patients from relatives' grief
        144–5
    therapeutic emplotment 143

families, of newly diagnosed patients,
    research study
  aim 138
  approach 138–9
  background 137–8
  benefits and risks of research 141
  discussion 148–9
  findings 142–8
  helper therapy principle 141
  interviews 139, 141, 142
  previous research 138
  process 139–40
  researcher and power balance 140
  sample 139
fatigue
  several possible causes 226
  side-effect of chemotherapy 225–6
  see also somnolence syndrome
fatigue from chemotherapy, research
    study
  aggregated and mean scores 240–2
  data collection diary 229–30, 242–3
  design 227–8
  discussion 242–3
  fatigue times 233, 234–40
  mean scores by visual analogue scale
    241
  purpose 227
  rationale 226
  response rate 230
  results 230–42
  sample 231, 242
  time plot themes 230, 232, 234
  time plots by treatment protocol 233
  time plots by visual analogue scale
    235–6, 238–9
fungating malignant wounds
  antiseptics 215
  cleansing agents 215
  clinical significance 212–14
  conclusions 217–18
  development of 207–8
  dressings 210–12, 215-16. 218
  incidence and prevalence 209–10
  low research priority 213, 214, 217
  moist wound healing 215, 216–17

  odour prevention 213, 216
  palliative treatments 208–9, 217
  physical and psychological distress
    210–12
  presentation 208–9
  previous studies 209–17
  research questions 218–19
  sites of 207–8
  symptom control priorities 217
  tumour vasculature, hypoxia and tissue
    necrosis 208
  wet to dry regimes 215

general practitioners (GPs), fundholding
    97–8
government policy documents 97, 100
  see also Health of the Nation
GPs (general practitioners), fundholding
    97–8
hair loss, review of research (1989–1994)
    13, 15
health checks, for older adults 118, 119
Health of the Nation (White Paper)
  cancer targets 104–5
  and primary health care 113
  raising awareness of prevention methods
    120
health technology 105
helper therapy principle 141
holism, in the hospice movement 157–8
hospices
  attitude to death 152–3
  care for families and patients 158
  commitment to education 54, 55
  holism 157–8
  hospice as family 155–6
  hospice culture 53–6
  ideals influencing nurse–patient
    relationship 155
  knowing the patient 156–7
  links with community 53–4
  Macmillan Nurse Tutors in 53–6
  some resistance to change 55–6
  staff employment and personal
    bereavement 152
  support networks 54–5

time availability 158-9
use of touch 158
working environment 53–6
see also palliative care
Hospital Anxiety and Depression Scale 191,
    196, 197
information
    for black and minority ethnic groups
    88, 89–90, 92, 93
    for patients, review of research
    (1989–1994) 14, 15
insider research 31
involvement, in palliative care
    institutional 155–9
    interpersonal 159–62
    nurses' need for support 162
isolation, of specialist nurses 250

job satisfaction 34
    breast care nurses 30, 34, 41–2

language, black and minority ethnic groups
    92
lung cancer
    check-up guidelines 119
    clinical practice 106–7
    government targets 104
    mortality rates 106
    palliative care 107
    prevention 106
    screening 106
    and smoking 106

Macmillan Nurse Tutors (MNTs)
    aim of role 49
    autonomy of, in hospices 54
    and colleges of nursing 56–63
    funding of posts 49, 64
    in the hospice environment 53–6
    and market philosophy 64
    multi-faceted role 64
    and organisational structure 53
Macmillan Nurse Tutors (MNTs), research
    study
    aim 49
    background 49–50

discussion 63-4
interviews 50, 52
methods 50
role sets 51
sample 50, 52–3
Macmillan nurses, *see* Cancer Relief
    Macmillan Fund; Macmillan Nurse
    Tutors; Paediatric Macmillan Nurses
mammography screening 125
mastectomies 199–200
minority ethnic groups, *see* black and
    minority ethnic groups
MNTs, *see* Macmillan Nurse Tutors
moist wound healing theory (MWHT) 215,
    216–17
morbidity, *see* psychological morbidity
MWHT (moist wound healing theory) 215,
    216–17

National Breast Screening Programme
    107–8, 189–90
National Health Service, changes in
    97–8
needs, assessment of, review of
    research (1989–1994) 11–12, 14,
    15
networking, breast care nurses 38
NHS, *see* National Health Service
nurses
    role of, reports and recommendations
    102–3
    roles and communication, review of
    research (1989–1994) 7–9
    see also breast care nurses; cancer
    nurses; palliative care nurses; staff's
    opinions and roles.
nursing records
    in breast care nursing 40, 44
    UKCC guidelines 40

Older adults
    health checks 118, 119
    influences on health beliefs 123–6
    knowledge of early signs 114, 126–7,
    128
    promoting cancer awareness in 126–0

reluctance to report symptoms 114–15, 124
see also early detection
oncology nurses, *see* cancer nurses
oncology services, *see* cancer services
oral assessment guides, review of research (1989–1994) 12, 15

Paediatric Macmillan nurses 69
Paediatric Oncology Outreach Nurse Specialists (POONSs
    'boundary crossing' role 75, 76
    characteristics of 68
    in different health care settings 75–6
    doctors' views of 72
    emotional labour 77–8
    funding 68
    growth in number of posts 68
    need for flexibility 74–5
    parents' views of 71–3
    professional network 68
    reasons for inception of service 68
    role challenges 73–8
    role of 71–3
    sensitivity to individual needs 74–5
    working with other professionals 72, 73, 76, 78
Paediatric Oncology Outreach Nurse Specialists (POONSs), research study
    background 67–9
    conclusions 78
    interviews 69
    methods 69
    sample 69–70
paediatrics, *see* children; Paediatric Oncology Outreach Nurse Specialists
palliative care
    black and minority ethnic groups 83–5, 85–6
    definition 85, 109, 212
    EAGC report 110
    goal of 85
    institutional involvement in 155–9
    interpersonal involvement in 159–62
    lung cancer 107
    for non-cancer patients 85
    settings for 109
    statistics 110
    see also hospices
palliative care, nurses and involvement in, research study
    background literature 151–3
    conclusions 162–3
    design and methods 153–4
    findings and discussion 155–62
    interviews 153–4
    sample 153–4
palliative care nurses
    dimensions of role 156
    and personal bereavement 151–2, 159–63
Person-Environment Fit Model of Occupational Stress 151–2
physical problems, review of research (1989–1994)
    assessment of needs 11–12, 15
    treatments 13,15
POONSs, *see* Paediatric Oncology Outreach Nurse Specialists
Post-Registration Education and Practice (PREP) 49
prevention
    awareness and lack of awareness of need 118, 120
    government initiatives 104
    lung cancer 106
    need for nurse training in 120
    and patients' educational levels 125
    review of research (1989–1994) 16, 17
    role confusion in services 122
    role of primary health care team 113
    skin cancer 109
primary health care, role in prevention 113
Project 2000 49, 56
prostate cancer
    awareness of need for prevention 118
    check-up guidelines 119
psychological morbidity with breast cancer
    mastectomy not the cause? 199
    need for reassurance 199
    style of consultation 198, 199

symptomatic *v.* screen-detected cancer 190, 201
psychological morbidity with breast cancer, research study
    conclusions 201–2
    discussion 196, 198–201
    interviews 193–6, 197
    methods 191
    results 193–6, 197
    sample 191, 192, 194
    standardised measures 191, 193
purchasing authorities 97–8

Quality of Life scales, review of research (1989–1994) 11, 12

racism
    and access to services 84, 93–4
    experiencing 91, 94
radiotherapy, reports and recommendations 101
records, *see* nursing records
reflexivity, definition 153
rehabilitation, review of research (1989–1994) 8, 9
religion, black and minority ethnic groups 90–1
repression 169, 180
research
    combined methods in 31, 251
    insider research 31
    methodology 18–21
    review of (1989–1994) 1–17
    summary of (1989–1994) 17-18
    see also subjects of specific studies
Rotterdam Symptom Checklist 193
Royal College of Nursing, Breast Care Nursing Society 29, 38

scalp cooling, review of research (1989–1994) 13, 15
screening 105
    age-related trend in offers of 114
    cervical cancer 108
    lack of awareness as constraint on 118–19
lung cancer 106
male attitudes to 126
mammography 125
underscreening of older adults 114
    see also breast screening; *and under* cervical cancer; lung cancer
Self-Esteem Linear Analogue Scale (SES) 193
services, assessment of, review of research (1989–1994) 2, 3–5, 7
SES, *see* Self-Esteem Linear Analogue Scale
signs, *see* symptoms and signs
Sixteen Personality Factor Questionnaire 34
skin cancer
    check-up guidelines 119
    government target 105, 109
    prevention 109
SMAC (Standing Medical Advisory Committee) report 98–9, 100–2
smoking
    government targets 104
    and lung cancer 104, 106
somnolence syndrome
    review of research (1989–1994) 10, 11
    see also fatigue
specialist nurses
    clinical nurse specialists 29, 40–1
    isolation of 250
staff's opinions and roles
    review of research (1989–1994) 6, 7–9
    see also nurses
Standing Medical Advisory Committee (SMAC) report 98–9, 100–2
stress
    nurses' views, review of research (1989–1994) 6, 7
    Person–Environment Fit Model of Occupational Stress 151–2
surgery, reports and recommendations 101
symptoms and signs
    older people's reluctance to report 114–15, 124

syringe drivers, review of research
    (1989–1944) 13, 15

therapeutic employment 143
therapeutic sensibility 167
touch, use of, in hospices 158

training *see* education and training
treatment, review of research (1989–1994)
    13, 15
triangulation 31

wounds, *see* fungating malignant wounds